Core Surgical
Training Interviews

Core Surgical Training Interviews

An A-Z Guide

Sukhpreet Singh Dubb

MBBS (Hons) BSc (Hons) BDS (Hons) MRCS

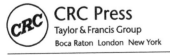

CRC Press
Taylor & Francis Group
Boca Raton London New York

CRC Press is an imprint of the
Taylor & Francis Group, an **informa** business

by CRC Press
Taylor & Francis Group
6000 Broken Sound Parkway NW, Suite 300
Boca Raton, FL 33487-2742

International Standard Book Number-13: 978-0-3674-3750-3 (Hardback)
978-0-3674-2737-5 (Paperback)

Library of Congress Cataloging-in-Publication Data

Names: Dubb, Sukhpreet Singh, author.
Title: Core surgical training interviews : an A-Z guide / Sukhpreet Dubb.
Description: First edition. | Boca Raton : CRC Press, 2020. | Includes bibliographical references and index. | Summary: "Each year the competition ratio for UK Core Surgical Training jobs is high. For every 3.3 applicants, only one will be successfully appointed to a CST post. This revision guide maximises the chances of interview success by providing comprehensive application and interview advice. Chapters include Clinical, Portfolio and Management stations and include both advice and real clinical scenarios, enabling trainee surgeons to save time and gain interview confidence"-- Provided by publisher.
Identifiers: LCCN 2020020120 (print) | LCCN 2020020121 (ebook) | ISBN 9780367437503 (hardback) | ISBN 9780367427375 (paperback) | ISBN 9781003005490 (ebook)
Subjects: MESH: General Surgery--education | Education, Medical, Graduate | Interviews as Topic | Job Application | United Kingdom | Study Guide
Classification: LCC RD37.2 (print) | LCC RD37.2 (ebook) | NLM WO 18.2 | DDC 617.0076--dc23
LC record available at https://lccn.loc.gov/2020020120
LC ebook record available at https://lccn.loc.gov/2020020121

Visit the Taylor & Francis Web site at
http://www.taylorandfrancis.com

and the CRC Press Web site at
http://www.crcpress.com

Typeset in Helvetica
by Nova Techset Private Limited, Bengaluru & Chennai, India

To every teacher who looked beyond where I came from and nurtured instead what I

could become. To every mentor who helped me focus on treading

the road ahead.

CONTENTS

FOREWORD

Preparing for and then attending a professional interview can be daunting. In UK surgery selection, interviews take place nationally for both core (basic surgical) and then for the higher (specialty) training. In recent years, the core surgery interview has become more akin to an objective structured clinical examination (OSCE). It is therefore much harder to impress the assessors with one's panache and personality. The best way to perform well and to maximise the chance of success is by careful planning and preparation.

This book written by Sukhpreet Singh Dubb – a recent core trainee and current specialty trainee in oral and maxillofacial surgery (OMFS) – provides an excellent and much needed resource for doctors attending the core surgery training (CST) interview. Following an excellent introduction providing an overview of the process, including the criteria used for selection, the chapter on interview skills helps candidates to improve and polish their technique. Subsequent chapters include audit, CV and discussion of the common scenario-type questions and skills that regularly appear in the interview process.

There is no doubt that this book should be essential reading for doctors approaching the CST interview, and I am confident that the book will gain rapid success.

Peter A Brennan MD, PhD, FRCS, Hon FRCS, FFST RCS, FDSRCS
Past Chair, RCS England Court of Examiners and Intercollegiate Committee for Basic
Surgical Examinations (MRCS and DOHNS)
Consultant oral and maxillofacial surgeon
Honorary Professor of Surgery
Queen Alexandra Hospital
Portsmouth PO6 3LY UK

PREFACE

Core surgical training represents an invaluable introduction into formalised surgical training. It is an opportunity to either discover new surgical specialties or confirm prior aspirations for a particular field. Candidates can tailor this period of training to explore various surgical specialties or combine allied surgical fields to complement their ambitions. For many core surgical trainees, this is a training period in which they will have greater responsibility for managing surgical presentations in the emergency setting, develop decision-making in clinics and expand their surgical skillset within theatres.

This book aims to provide a comprehensive overview of the interview stations but also the thinking process and logical steps behind surgical presentations, investigations, diagnosis and management. I wish every reader the greatest success and hope this book helps on your journey in entering the world of surgery.

ACKNOWLEDGEMENTS

I would like to thank Dr Ashley Ferro MB, BChir, BSc (Hons) for his help with this book.

AUTHOR

Dr Sukhpreet Singh Dubb is dual-qualified as a surgeon and dentist, and is training to be a consultant in facial surgery. He is the author of a number of successful medical revision guides. He has authored over 50 publications, presentations and posters in leading journals and conferences, and has been awarded more than 20 prizes for international research, academic and leadership activities. He was also the UK ambassador at the White House and United Nations and was invited to speak at the House of Commons as a champion for widening participation. He also acts as a non-executive director and advisor to technology companies using blockchain and telemedicine technology.

1. INTRODUCTION

1.1 INTRODUCTION

Core surgical training (CST) is a two-year programme formalising and providing a foundation within the general principles of surgery that also allows for themed subspecialty content, thus suiting the needs and aspirations of successful candidates.

Prior to this centralised process, trainees would often spend several years informally applying and training in surgical specialties that interested them, without any formal basis, to ensure they met the foundation requirements of the CST pathway. National recruitment started in 2013 with a centralised and formal process. This aims to ensure a fair process and provides candidates with a wide range of surgical specialties and geographical locations to train in. Since, applications, communication regarding interviews and the outcomes of interviews are published through an online system.

Although CST represents the first formal step into beginning your surgical training, make no mistake, the very best candidates will start their preparations well in advance of the application process. You must remain focused, organised and able to act quickly to address any weaknesses in your candidacy. This book aims to focus your efforts and ensure you leave no stone unturned in securing the very best score possible in your applications.

> ...make no mistake, the very best candidates will start their preparations well in advance of the application process. You must remain focused, organised and able to act quickly to address any weaknesses in your candidacy.

All applicants must meet the essential criteria in order to be listed for interviews; currently these include:

- GMC registration and licence to practise
- Foundation competences. Usually this is achieved by completing a UK Foundation Programme within 3 years of the intended start date. An applicant can also submit alternative evidence by asking a consultant who has supervised them for at least 3 months to attest to their achievement of foundation competency
- Advanced Life Support (ALS) course completed by the intended start date
- Less than 18 months of surgical experience

The structure of national interviews

Although the structure and process of CST national interviews have been constantly reviewed since 2013, there have been three scoring stations: Clinical scenario, management and portfolio themed stations. Each of these stations lasts 10 minutes, with a break between stations. Pilot stations have been introduced in the past that have no bearing on your final score. Each station tends to have two surgical consultant interviewers, typically not related to the scenario that is being asked; for example, you will not necessarily have a set of orthopaedic consultants asking you an orthopaedic-themed clinical scenario.

Places are offered based upon a cutoff score that determines if you are 'appointable' or not. Candidates who score above this cutoff score (this changes every year) are then offered a training programme position depending on their score and choice ranking. Successful candidates are currently given 48 hours to accept, reject or hold their offer. They may also apply for an upgrade if a more preferable training position becomes available.

Be prepared!

You should start the following steps prior to the advertised opening date of applications:

1. Write a comprehensive 'long CV' (see next section) that includes your every achievement since you started medical school. This will guide you easily through your application form, help you answer self-assessment questions and aid the planning of your portfolio. **More importantly** the long CV should quickly identify areas that are clearly your strengths, areas that require some improvement and, vitally, your areas of weakness;

2. Begin accumulating your vital documents early such as passport, GMC certificate, foundation competences and appropriate visa and English proficiency documents. For each of these you will need multiple photocopies, all of which is time consuming. Without these you can be long-listed out of the process at any stage, or fail to achieve marks for achievements due to lack of evidence;

3. Prepare your reading materials to address each of the three stations in the interview. For you, this is easy, as everything you need – including ample practice stations – is in this guide!

4. We strongly recommend finding an interview partner or a small group of 2–3 in order to practise the various interview scenarios. Much of your time will be spent accumulating the appropriate knowledge and training yourself to think and answer typical interview questions. However, leading up to the interview itself, face-to-face interviews in our experience are invaluable. Use the scenarios and questions in this guide with your colleagues to polish your interview demeanour and style; and

5. Finally, split your activities into 'active' and 'inactive'. Gathering and printing your portfolio documents is an important activity but is time consuming and 'inactive'. In contrast, completing the loop of an audit to include in your portfolio and practising interview scenarios are 'active' processes that will directly aid your application into CST. You must allocate more time towards your activities that are active and, where possible, reduce those that are inactive.

The long CV

The following are suggested headings for your long CV, some of the important areas you should identify. We will expand on all of these areas later in the guide. This will help with your application form, as well as your portfolio. **Note this is not how your final portfolio will appear but allows you to collate the evidence of your application as well as an overview of your surgical-oriented career so far.**

1. Employment

Foundation training posts, specialties and supervisors. Rank your most recent posts first.

2. Academic

MBBS, BSc, all distinctions, honours and merit details, MRCS, etc.

3. **Honours and prizes**

   For example, academic, extracurricular, national/international prizes, etc.

4. **Publications**

   For example, only fully accepted/press articles indexed by PubMed. Rank your first-authorship papers first.

5. **Oral presentations**

   Rank presentations in chronological order, and highlight your name in bold.

6. **Posters**

   Rank presentations in chronological order, and highlight your name in bold.

7. **Audit experience**

   List all projects – and most importantly those where you have closed the loop.

8. **Elective**

   Prepare any outcomes from the elective such as reports and experiences.

9. **Leadership experience**

   Formal courses and activities that supplement leadership.

10. **Teaching experience**

    Formal teaching experiences.

11. **Courses**

    This will include BSS, ATLS, CCrISP, etc.

12. **eLogbook**

    Surgical eLogbook as well as selected parts of your NHS portfolio assessments.

Vertical and horizontal domains

It can be very easy to mistake the CST process as simply three stand-alone stations (clinical, management and portfolio). '**Vertical domains**' are tested in these stations, that is domains that test how much knowledge you have on a specific topic, for example dealing with upper gastrointestinal bleeding in the clinical station, dealing with difficult colleagues in the management station, and so forth. However, there are also important '**horizontal domains**' that are present and tested across all three stations, for example verbal and non-verbal communication skills.

Many candidates do not fully appreciate or understand the new role they are applying for and therefore structure their approach for the interviews inadequately by concentrating on vertical domains only. You must bring a level of maturity to the CST interview that can be seen in your seniors – not only when dealing with an acute presentation, but also in the important teamwork and administration that is involved in safely transferring patients from the emergency department into theatres.

The following are the horizontal domains you should combine with your long CV; ensure that you can fill each of the categories with evidence – work-based assessments, courses and achievements. We have given some examples of the evidence you can use to support each domain. We have incorporated these horizontal domains in all of the example stations within this book.

Education and Teaching
- Variable teaching methodology
- Range of teaching audiences
- Planned formal teaching sessions that involve assessments

Evidence: Planned teaching, teaching courses, teaching feedback, teaching timetables

Management
- Leadership skills
- Team-working skills
- Quality and safety improvements

Evidence: Clinical governance, leadership courses

Clinical Practice
- Clinical judgement
- Patient assessment
- Documentation
- Infection control
- Patient safety

Evidence: Work-based assessments

Promoting Good Health
- Understand important health policies for patients
- Appreciate chronic care patients and self-care
- Evidence of reducing the burden of disease in the community
- Removing inequalities in the standard and provision of health care

Evidence: Contribution to public health articles, extracurricular/humanitarian activities

Communication Skills
- Patient communication
- Colleague communication
- Breaking bad news

Evidence: Assessment of communication skills during interview questioning

Research and Training
- Evidence of research
- Understand the importance of guidelines
- Audit cycles
- Evidence of personal development

Evidence: Portfolio evidence

Ethics and probity
- Understanding legal frameworks in medicine
- Consent
- Confidentiality
- Medical ethics
- Medical error and integrity

Evidence: Assessed during interview questions

We are delighted that you have invested in this guide, and hope that the advice and scenarios given within help you make the best application possible to begin your surgical career. Throughout, we have included feedback and insights from past candidates who share their experiences. We hope that this knowledge and these insights help you learn from their mistakes – but also gain from their success.

1.2 INTERVIEW SKILLS

1. Communication skills
2. Using a system: SALE, SCAM and SCAPE
3. Applying the system

As practitioners, our daily routine involves displaying exemplary communication skills in order to best aid our patients. The skills needed in taking a focused history, or presenting findings to a senior are not dissimilar to those under scrutiny by the interviewers. Your communication skills deserve as much attention as reviewing common interview questions and refreshing your knowledge base. The interviewers will examine your response to pressure, not only in terms of the answers you give, but the manner that you react to them. We have mentioned systems and structures to aid your verbal communication, next are the non-verbal skills you should maintain at all times during your interview preparation and also examples from past candidates of their importance.

Appearance, gestures, facial expressions and eye contact

The importance of appearing immaculate and professional is obvious, however, you must simultaneously be comfortable during the interview in order to perform optimally. Be organised and have your clothes prepared well in advance; closer to the interview dates, wear your clothes and practise in them, if they are new. Ensure that whatever you wear, you are comfortable. Do not forget about polishing your shoes or ensuring you have ironed your clothes if you are staying in accommodation the day before the interview. As the interview dates approach these obvious actions are easily overlooked and easily forgotten.

> During the management station I was asked to clarify my answer about venous thrombosis prophylaxis and how seriously I would pursue a situation where it was not being administered. This was my first challenging question, and before I had realised, I noticed I was frowning and rubbing my forehead. I had made it obvious to the interviewer how unsure I was. In the next station, I focused on keeping a more neutral, professional appearance, and even though the questions were harder it went much more smoothly.

Body positioning and spatial distance

In most stations, there will be a table in between you and the interviewers. In the portfolio station, this allows your portfolio to be displayed, but also the examiners will have their mark sheets and papers in front of them. Practise a professional and comfortable body position and be aware at all times of your spatial behaviours, such as hand movements. This is particularly helpful when you are collecting your thoughts before answering a question and particularly vital when challenged.

Tone and pace of voice

Do not become disheartened when you begin your revision and practice. As you progress through this guide, you will find that your knowledge increases exponentially along with the other domains. You must remember that precision and accuracy, rather than quantity, are more important. Ensure you practise and critique your answers not only in their content, but also in the manner of their delivery.

> My clinical station was the worst across the three. I did well with the clinical scenario but then the other interviewer asked me about airway management

and I started to just babble. When you don't know an answer it's better to just say so, and move onto something else or take a moment to think. It's defensive and natural to say something when you're not sure. This, I felt, then took away from the good answers that I did give.

The less obvious interview practice techniques are just as important and they go a long way. I had a bad habit of tapping my feet and wringing my hands when I was thinking or there was a difficult question. I spent time just practising to keep my hands and feet together, and asking my friends and family to ask me normal questions. I also practised questions with my colleagues once I felt more confident. During the interview, I felt much more composed and consistent. A lot of my friends lost their composure under the pressure, and without actively practising, it's very easy to fall apart on the day. This seems blindingly obvious but don't underestimate the pressure you will be under during the interview!

Using a system

Using simple principles to answer questions can be invaluable during the interview as it also provides consistency when practising particular stations. Next we have given three different styles of questions and some mnemonics to include in your arsenal when tackling these questions.

Broad-based, generalised questioning

'After core-surgical training what would you like to accomplish in 5 years? 10 years? 20 years?'

In response to a broad topic that aims to cover multiple topics use '**SALE**'

Surgical	(Career and clinical accomplishments)
Academic	(Teaching and educational goals)
Leadership	(Managerial roles)
Extracurricular	(Social and family-orientated activities)

Acute situation or presentation questioning

'How would you manage a patient who has suffered an abdominal wound dehiscence?'

In response to more acute topics use '**SCAM**'

Scenario	(Identify the most important and relevant information available)
Context	(Place the situation into the full background of events)
Appraisal	(Assess the available options and appropriate responses)
Management	(Formulation of a management plan)

Complicated or ethical situation

'How would you deal with a senior registrar taking an illicit substance in the doctor's mess?'

In response to more in-depth or complex topics use '**SCAPE?**'

Scenario	(Identify the most important and relevant information available)
Context	(Place the situation into the full background of events)
Appraisal	(Assess the available options and appropriate responses)
Prioritise	(This usually encompasses patient safety)
Escalate	(Once the limit of your influence is reached, activate senior/appropriate support)

Applying the system

Each of your surgical interviews lasts 10 minutes. The number of questions that may be posed is very variable, and this is often dependent on the methodology of your answers. In our experience, rather than depth, we have noticed the examiners to ask a series of questions in all of the stations. You must therefore execute each question with precision and accuracy and limit any irrelevant material. The previous section has given you a structure for answering questions, we now outline a general pro forma which you should apply to every answer you give.

Listen CAREFULLY to the examiner and answer the question

Time and again in examinations and interviews you will come across this mantra, however, do not gloss over this simple but important principle. In the 2013 interview, a candidate was asked how to determine if a patient who had vomited and discarded the contents may have had haematemesis. The trainee focused on regurgitating as much knowledge they had on haematemesis and its management, rather than the more relevant details of examining the patient for blood on their lips and clothing, appearance of pallor, shortness of breath, inserting a nasogastric tube to simultaneously relieve vomiting and examine the gastric contents, and so on. This is the most common error in interviews and examinations, and we urge you to remain vigilant against it.

> *In the 2013 interview, a candidate was asked how to determine if a patient who had vomited and discarded the contents may have had haematemesis. The trainee focused on regurgitating as much knowledge they had on haematemesis and its management, rather than the more relevant details.*

Utilise a system

We have given an example of systems used to give structure to your answers. There are many others, practise each of your questions to ensure you convey an efficient, well-thought-out answer. The advantage of using the SALE, SCAM and SCAPE system is that it formulates your answer on a principle rather than encouraging you to memorise information. Following this system will ensure your answers are well structured without sounding too rehearsed.

Time management

This is perhaps the most difficult skill to practise, as it is dependent upon the question you have been asked. However, as the examiners tend to ask a series of questions based on a theme – diagnosis, investigation, management of a patient with an aneurysm – we suggest limiting each of your answers to between 90 seconds and 2 minutes. Your interview practice will likely grossly exceed this; however, practise regularly to reduce your answers to the most relevant principles and facts.

2. INTRODUCTION TO THE CLINICAL STATIONS

The clinical interview station represents a significant challenge, and in our review of past trainees, it is consistently the most daunting of the three stations due to the breadth of knowledge needed. The interviewers tend to follow a theme and this will be based on the clinical vignette that you are presented with, whilst another examiner asks you other related questions. You must simultaneously present a calm, competent and professional demeanor whilst constructing and communicating accurate, precise and well-structured answers.

> *During my clinical station one interviewer focused mainly on the vignette for which I had time to think and was able to answer most questions, the other interviewer asked me completely different questions. I had completed lower GI and orthopaedic rotations but the interviewer asked me a topic in ENT. Even during medical school, I hadn't been exposed to a great deal of ENT and had no clinical experience in it. I went back to basic principles and thought what I would do to ensure I was being as safe as possible.*

The clinical questions are based upon the common presentations that you would encounter whilst on-call as a surgical trainee, as well as the common elective surgical pathologies. Do not panic and begin revising all of your surgical final notes. The interviewers are not looking for memorised factual detail, they wish to see you think in a logical, safe and competent manner that makes you appropriate for further surgical teaching and training.

2.1 ABSCESS

Clinical Case

A 24-year-old male complains of an offensive foul-smelling discharge from his natal cleft area. The problem first started with a boil that burst without any intervention. On examination, the patient has widely distributed dense hair.

Describe the clinical photograph. What is the pathology shown?

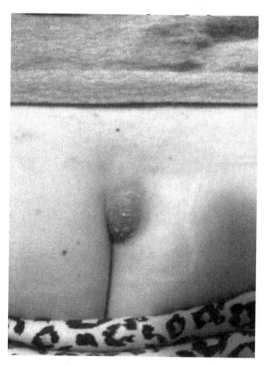

> This is an example of a vertical learning domain where you are expected to demonstrate your knowledge of a given topic. The interviewer will question your ability to think logically, safely and competently.

This is a clinical photograph depicting a patient's gluteal region. There is an oval-shaped erythematous lesion in the upper medial aspect of the patient's right gluteal muscle close to the natal cleft. The lesion is well demarcated with raised borders. There appears to be multiple droplets on the surface of the lesion representing exudate, but no obvious punctum or gross discharge is visible. The surrounding skins appears largely disease free. This clinical photograph is in keeping with an active pilonidal abscess.

What is an abscess?

This is a localised collection of pus which is usually encased within granulation tissue. The disease process involves the exponential increase of by-products, secondary to the action of enzymes, released from polymorphs and macrophages. These products accumulate causing an increase in the osmotic pressure and therefore size of the abscess. The expansion occurs along fascial lines that provide the least degree

> As you execute each question, they will become progressively more challenging. Do not worry if you see advanced questions in this guide – the principle is to challenge you to think and apply knowledge.

of resistance, until eventually the abscess bursts. This is usually into a hollow viscus, a cavity such as the peritoneum, or commonly the external environment via skin or mucous membranes.

How would you treat a pilonidal abscess?

In the acute setting, I would treat a pilonidal abscess as any other abscess with an incision and drainage procedure under general anaesthetic. I would first resuscitate the patient and assess their level of health using the ALS protocol A, B, C. I would then take a focused history and ascertain important details such as their last meal, important medical diseases such as diabetes, use of steroids and if they smoke. I would then examine the abscess itself, as I have described.

On examination, what features would you be looking for in a pilonidal abscess?

On examination, I would specifically look for evidence of pits within the midline and surrounding lateral tracks. The presence of an asymptomatic midline pit pathology, without surrounding satellite tracks, suggests mild disease and conservative management can be offered. This includes meticulous hygiene of the area and regular depilation. In symptomatic disease and in the presence of lateral tracts, surgical intervention should be considered. The intervention types are varied, the principle depends on the presence of infection. If an infection is present, laying open the tracts and allowing granulation to occur is preferred, whilst in clean wounds, primary closure can be attempted. I would always inform the patient that despite infection-free appearing wounds, the primary closure can still fail. Other variations and approaches also exist such as the Bascom and Karydakis procedures.

What is the Karydakis procedure?

This is one of several procedures that attempts primary closure of the wound site. Typically, an asymmetric elliptical incision is created with the larger area of the incision encompassing the lateral tracts. Undermining of the skin helps to create a flap that moves the wound away from midline without creating tension, which would inhibit healing. The dissection then proceeds to the level of the pre-sacral fascia in order to remove as many potential tracts as possible.

What factors could contribute towards recurrent pilonidal disease?

Recurrence is an unfortunate risk that I would warn my patients about when consenting or explaining procedures for removal. During surgery, part of the lesion may have been missed, despite incision down to the level of the pre-sacral fascia. Part of the postoperative process is scrupulous hygiene and shaving of the area. Unfortunately, new hairs can re-enter through the skin, or even the new scar tissue. Finally, the midline wound may be created by shearing along planes and incomplete scar formation. This creates a new potential cavity for disease processes to return to.

Background Information

There are usually two examiners in the clinical station, with variation in the format of the interview, however, most trainees reiterate that one examiner focuses on the clinical vignette and a discussion around this whilst the other can pose varied questions. This can be on a new vignette, a single chosen topic or indeed questions at random.

A pilonidal sinus results from the forceful protrusion of hair fibres through the skin, creating a subcutaneous sinus. This most commonly occurs at the natal cleft in the sacrococcygeal area. There is a resultant chronic inflammatory reaction and multiple sinuses can potentially communicate through a single deep cavity. The inflammatory process presents with discharge and there is risk of subsequent abscess formation. The disease can be debilitating and commonly affects young men. It has a preponderance in hirsute individuals with loose stiff hairs alongside skin that is broken or macerated. Chronic trauma can allow hair tips to penetrate the skin whilst the rolling motion of the buttock area encourages deep burrowing of the hair strands. Typically, occupations affected are those involving prolonged seating, hairdressers and sheep-shearers (particularly in between finger webs). Other locations outside the perianal area include the axilla and umbilicus. Important features to elicit from the history include pain, swelling and discharge from the sacrococcygeal area. Diagnosis is based upon clinical examination with the presence of midline pits and sinus tracts, or complication by abscess formation.

In asymptomatic patients, local hair removal through shaving or laser therapy is encouraged alongside hygiene of the affected area. Symptomatic patients with no abscess formation should undergo surgical intervention; currently there is no dominance between primary closure (which heals faster but suffers from increased recurrence) or healing via secondary intention. A discussion with the patient should be pursued to formulate the most ideal management. When primary closure is attempted, incisions in the midline should be avoided since they have higher recurrence and complication rates. Alongside surgery, prophylactic antibiotic therapy is often offered and depilation through laser therapy is recommended (shaving appears to increase recurrence rates). Lastly, in patients suffering from abscess formation, an incision and drainage procedure should be performed and healing followed by secondary intention alongside antibiotic cover and analgesic. In recurrent disease, a repeat of first line management is offered in both situations. More complex surgical techniques are often employed to compensate for the removal of midline tissues.

Important Terms:

Bascom's procedure: This involves a lateral incision to the midline, gaining entry to the sinus cavity. Removal of enclosed hair, debris and granulation tissue is performed, and finally excision and closure of the midline pits. The lateral wound allows drainage and is left to heal by secondary intention.

> *For the clinical station, I went through some surgery theory and practised as many scenarios with my friends. You have 2 minutes to study the vignette, which is valuable for organising your thoughts around the topics and questions that may arise. However, during the station the other interviewer interposed other questions in between my answers to the vignette. They were often completely different to the subject area of the vignette and after answering them the other interviewer took me back to a topic on the vignette. Answering a difficult question before returning to the vignette can break the momentum and flow of your thinking. Also focusing too much on the vignette can close your mind to the other topics that you can get asked. Lots of scenarios is my advice!*

2.2 ACUTE ABDOMEN I

Clinical Case

You are the surgical CT1 on call and you are referred a 20-year-old female presenting with a 24-hour history of acute lower abdominal pain. The pain started abruptly whilst watching TV and was shortly followed by nausea. She rates the pain as 10/10 and this is now mostly on the right side of her abdomen. She denies diarrhoea, dysuria or a recent travel history, but admits complete loss of appetite. She usually experiences painful menses lasting 1–2 days, and her last menstrual period was 7 days ago. She is on an oral contraceptive pill and denies any drug allergies. She is sexually active with a single partner, and is a non-smoker with occasional social alcohol intake.

Her observations are: BP: 130/90 mmHg; HR: 90; RR: 18; Temp: 38.3°C; Sats: 100% on air.

'What are your differentials?'

My primary diagnosis from this patient's presentation would be acute appendicitis. The acute nature of the presentation alongside characteristic features such as nausea, loss of appetite and migration of pain to the right iliac fossa as well as the patient's age group support this diagnosis. The differentials I would consider would include ectopic pregnancy, urinary tract infection, ovarian cyst pathology, pelvic inflammatory disease, Meckel's diverticulitis and inflammatory bowel disease. In order to support my primary diagnosis, I would like the opportunity to examine the patient.

'Describe the examination findings you would look for.'

For acute appendicitis on inspection, I would assess the discomfort and level of activity of the patient. I would examine for peripheral stigmata of disease to gauge the general health of the patient. At the abdomen, I would assess the patient for rigidity, area of maximal tenderness, typically over McBurney's point, as well as abdominal masses particularly over this landmark. I would see if Rovsing's sign was present. I would determine if the patient had any organomegaly, percuss the abdomen for signs of peritonism, tympanic sounds and also assess the presence of fluid through shifting dullness. Finally, I would auscultate for the presence of bowel sounds and perform a PR and PV examination in the presence of a chaperone.

'How would you manage this patient?'

I would resuscitate the patient and assess their level of health using the ALS protocol A, B, C. Once the patient is stable, I would conduct a full history and examination followed by investigations starting with bedside tests such as a urine dipstick and pregnancy test. I would then proceed to blood tests, ECG, chest radiographs and then more specialised investigations such as a CT scan, if indicated.

'Justify each of your investigations.'

A common structure employed when considering investigations is **SPUBEXS**. This proceeds from non-invasive bedside examinations, in a natural order, towards more invasive specialised investigations.

- – Sputum
- – Urine
- – Bloods
- – ECG
- – XR
- – Special investigations (ultrasound, CT, MRI, etc.)

Investigation	Explanation
Sputum	Sputum analysis for suspected chest infections, common in patients postoperatively. Not relevant in this particular patient.
Urine analysis	Haematuria, proteinuria, glucose, ketones, leukocytes, nitrites, specific gravity.
	Depending on the findings this can identify inflammatory conditions of the kidney, renal tract stones, diabetic ketoacidosis and urinary tract infections. A high yield, non-invasive test that is often missed. *Do not forget to perform a pregnancy test in appropriate patients.*
Bloods	FBC, urea and electrolytes, liver function tests, inflammatory markers, e.g. CRP, coagulation.
	Always mention the reason for each blood test selection e.g. FBC for raised WCC and neutrophils alongside raised CRP for supporting infective and inflammatory differentials.
ECG	Important in patients with co-morbidities, eliminating other differentials and also preparation of the patient for anaesthetic review if theatre is needed.
X-ray	This includes CXR and AXR. Erect CXR is mandatory in any patient with a suspected viscus perforation.
Special investigations	This includes ultrasound, ERCP, CT, MRI, etc.

'What diagnostic investigations would you consider?'

Investigation	Advantage	Disadvantage	Common Use
Ultrasound	Non-invasive, cheap and quick. Has a higher sensitivity and specificity for gynaecological pathology	Less useful for assessing appendix pathology, multiple factors such as body habitus and viscera can inhibit views	Young children, gynaecological pathology
CT	Accurately identifies appendiceal pathology	Exposure to radiation, can be falsely reassuring in early appendicitis	Suspected appendicitis, low consideration of gynaecological pathology
Diagnostic laparoscopy	Definitive assessment of appendix and surrounding organs	Involves a general anaesthetic and attending theatre	Uncertainty, or atypical presentations following investigations

'What diagnostic criteria is relevant for appendicitis?'

The MANTRELS score is a progressive score for appendicitis based upon clinical characteristics. The greater the score, the greater the chance of appendicitis.

M: Migration of pain to right lower quadrant	(1)
A: Anorexia	(1)
N: Nausea and vomiting	(1)
T: Tenderness in right lower quadrant	(2)
R: Rebound tenderness	(1)
E: Elevated temperature	(1)
L: Leukocytosis	(2)
S: Shift of WBC count to left	(1)

'What complications can occur in appendicitis?'

There are a number of important complications following an appendicitis. The most serious include perforation and subsequent generalised peritonitis. Perforation can occur as early as

12 hours after unremitting appendiceal inflammation. There is usually an acute deterioration in the patient's condition including fever, tenderness and reduced bowel sounds. This progresses to more generalised pain and absent bowel sounds. Delays in treatment can sometimes result in the formation of an appendiceal mass, or abscess, often palpable and tender on examination. This can be confirmed by US or CT scan, management is conservative with intravenous antibiotics and fluid resuscitation. An interval appendicectomy can be performed if there is not full resolution after 6 weeks.

Background Information

Appendicitis is among the commonest surgical presentations, with a slight male preponderence (1.3:1). It can be defined as the acute inflammation of the vermiform appendix, most commonly due to obstruction from a faecolith or infection causing lymphoid hyperplasia. Patients typically present with acute centralised abdominal pain which migrates to the right iliac fossa as diffuse visceral irritation transforms to more localised parietal peritoneal irritation. Important symptoms include fever, anorexia, nausea with or without vomiting and reduced bowel sounds. On examination, important signs to be aware of include:

Dunphy's sign: Increased pain with raised intra-abdominal pressure, for example coughing.

Rovsing's sign: Palpation or pressure in the left lower quadrant causes pain in the right lower quadrant.

Psoas sign: With the patient in the left lateral position, extension of the right hip causes pain in the right lower quadrant suggesting a retrocaecal appendix.

Obturator/Cope sign: Flexion and internal rotation of the right hip causes pain in the right lower quadrant if the appendix lies close to obturator internus.

Treatment is dependent on the state of the appendix, and if there are any complicating factors:

- Uncomplicated appendicitis: Appendicectomy with/without IV antibiotic adjunctive care
- Appendicitis and perforation: Resuscitation, IV antibiotics with/without appendicectomy
- Appendicitis with abscess formation: CT guided drainage with/without interval appendicectomy.

Important terms:

Chronic/recurrent appendicitis: This can occur in up to 5% of patients with appendicitis and most often results from antibiotic therapy in subclinical/early appendicitis whereby the inflammatory process does not fully resolve;

Mesenteric adenitis: More common in children, where a painful lymphadenopathy of the small bowel mesentery occurs following a viral infection. This can mimic an appendicitis but can be treated with supportive therapy alone; and

Interval appendicectomy: Treatment option for appendicitis complication with abscess formation. Antibiotic therapy is initiated to reduce sepsis with drainage of the abscess under CT guidance. If symptoms do not resolve an appendicectomy is performed after an interval of usually 6 weeks.

Clinical vignettes for further practise

1. A 17-year-old female presents with a 2-day history of right iliac fossa pain. She denies fever or any bowel symptoms but suffers from nausea. Her urine analysis, including pregnancy test and FBC, are normal.

2. A 21-year-old male presents with 48-hour history of colicky umbilical pain, which has now migrated to the right iliac fossa. He complains of fever, nausea and loss of appetite.

3. A 19-year-old female presents with increasing right iliac fossa pain, nausea and fever. She denies any PV discharge. On examination her abdomen is soft, diffusely tender in the suprapubic region with possible right adnexal tenderness.

> One of the most helpful exercise I did towards the end of my interview practice, once I had been through enough stations, was tangential learning. I would run through a clinical topic like appendicitis and then pick on subjects from my answer and expand on them, for example. Meckels' diverticulitis, blood investigations, consenting patients, etc. The experience of going through enough stations is that you can start to think through scenarios, and second-guess where interviewers are likely to ask you questions. Practise as many station scenarios as you can to reacquaint yourself with the clinical knowledge. I found it helpful to constantly think what I had seen my registrars doing – like phoning theatres and reviewing relevant test results. Perhaps the most important principle is to be safe, always think: What is the safest thing to do for my patient?

2.3 ACUTE ABDOMEN II

Clinical Case

You receive a call from A/E about a 44-year-old male who has presented with a 3-month history of on-going epigastric pain. They described the pain as constant and dull which often wakes them from their sleep. They have seen their GP who has prescribed ranitidine and omeprazole, however food and milk are the most relieving factors. The A/E doctor has called you because the patient has not responded to analgesic and is close to breaching.

'How would you proceed with this patient?'

Since this is a telephone referral from a colleague over the phone, I would enquire about more information in addition to the history. I would first ask how worried the clinician was about the patient and ask for the patient's observations including their blood pressure, heart rate, respiratory rate and oxygen saturations during the period of their presentation. I would also ask if the patient looked unwell or unstable. If I was satisfied that this wasn't an acutely unwell patient, I would then proceed to ask more details including any haematemesis, PR bleeding or malaena. I would ask for the patient's past medical and surgical history including any previous upper GI endoscopies and operations. Regarding their drug history, I would want to know the full repertoire of medications they take on a regular basis, the medications they had tried before presenting to A/E including NSAIDS. Whilst the patient had been in A/E, I would want to know the analgesic that had been offered and also if the patient was known to be allergic to any medication. Finally, I would ask about any heavy alcohol intake.

> Listen, listen and listen to the question posed! Here the candidate has not proceeded to state they would begin by resuscitating the patient. The vignette is clear in stating you are being referred a patient over the phone, and therefore gathering more information before you formally accept and see the patient demonstrates your maturity and experience.

'What would you do for the patient in the emergency department?'

I would begin by formally resuscitating the patient myself and assessing their level of health using the ALS protocol A, B, C. Once the patient is stable, I would conduct a full history and examination focusing on the abdominal system and measure basic observations, as I mentioned previously. I would then follow this with relevant investigations including urine dipstick, blood investigations, an ECG and erect CXR.

> As your experience in these scenarios increases you can begin to pre-empt the interviewers' questions. A common question is the alternative position if an erect CXR cannot be taken or if no free air excludes a perforation. Rather than wait to be asked this you can incorporate this into your answer. From an interviewer's perspective this is a mark of excellence.

'What are you looking for on the erect CXR?'

This patient has an acute abdomen and based on the history I would wish to exclude a visceral perforation. I would look for signs of a pneumoperitoneum by examining for air under the diaphragm and above the liver edge. If the patient was too unwell, I would ask the radiographer to position the patient in the left lateral decubitus position. Any free intra-abdominal air would therefore rise and present in between the liver and lateral abdominal wall. I would still consider other investigations if there was no free air under the diaphragm, as this can be missing in more than 30% of affected patients.

'Other than a viscus perforation, what else can cause free air under the diaphragm?'

The commonest cause for free air under the diaphragm is recent abdominal surgery, hence the importance of a past surgical history. Air is typically absorbed after 1 week following abdominal surgery, though this is much quicker in laparoscopic procedures. Other causes not relevant to this patient include ventilated patients or those suffering from chronic obstructive airways disease where gas escapes from the tracheobronchial tree. Vaginal examination or tubal insufflation in gynaecological investigations can also introduce air visible on an erect CXR. Finally, the interposition of a gas-filled viscus, such as the transverse colon between the liver and diaphragm, can appear as free gas and this is called Chilaiditi's sign.

'The following blood results appear for this patient; how would you proceed?'

Hb	12.0
MCV	80
WCC	9.0
Neutrophils	6.5
Sodium	140
Potassium	4.5
Urea	6.0
Creatinine	100
Bilirubin	10
ALT	30
AST	29
ALP	31

These blood results appear grossly normal; the only abnormality I can see is a normocytic anaemia which does support a diagnosis of peptic ulcer disease. My other differentials would include hypersplenism or acute blood loss, for example oesophageal varices or trauma. Renal failure can also cause a normocytic anaemia, but the renal function is normal in this patient.

'How would you manage this patient if your examination findings and investigations were normal?'

This patient appears to be suffering from abdominal pain which is most likely due to uncontrolled peptic ulcer disease. The patient has a normocytic anaemia but is otherwise stable, and I would first control his pain with appropriate analgesic, avoiding NSAID medication as this can precipitate a perforation. Once pain was controlled, I would discuss this patient and his investigations with my senior with a view to ensure he does not need acute surgical admission. I would suggest discharging the patient with pain relief and ask for the GP in the community to investigate the patient for *H. pylori* infection and, if positive, to treat this accordingly. I would organise an upper GI endoscopy procedure under the relevant team to ensure there were no worrying features overlooked by my acute investigations. Finally, I would explain this to the patient and provide them with a discharge summary, and any relevant patient information leaflets that may be available.

'Is it likely this patient has *H. pylori* infection if they are already being treated with PPIs?'

Proton-pump inhibitors, bismuth and antibiotics can interfere with the *H. pylori* test. Also, none of the investigations for *H. pylori*, including breath test or stool antigen tests, are

100% sensitive and it is reasonable to repeat these investigations in this patient – or more importantly, if an ulcer were to be found on endoscopy.

Background Information

Knowing when not to operate is a long-known adage which applies in this scenario designed to test your ability to recognise whether a patient needs an acute surgical admission. One could even state that the main clinical problem is one more suited for medical care; however, an acute abdomen will often be referred to surgical assessment first to eliminate important differentials. It is just as important to recognise and formulate conservative management plans as those requiring more active treatment.

Peptic ulcer disease arises from the imbalance of acid/pepsin production and protective measures such as the mucus barrier. The large majority of peptic ulcer disease is attributable to an *H. pylori* infection. Prior to this, management focused upon inhibiting the production of pepsin and acid through vagotomy, gastrectomy, H2 receptor antagonists and proton-pump inhibitors. *H. pylori* is a spiral, gram negative rod able to survive the gastric environment through potent urease activity, which produces ammonia and neutralises the acid around it. *H. pylori* can also directly damage mucosal membranes with protease activity causing subsequent inflammation.

There are five types of gastric ulcers. The most common is classified as type 1 presenting on the greater curvature of the stomach, where hypersecretion of acid and haemorrhage tend not to be causative factors. Conversely, type 2 ulcers are present in the same geographic location as type 1 ulcers, but are associated with excessive acid secretion and duodenal ulcer disease. The occurrence of haemorrhage, obstruction and perforation are much higher in type 2 ulcers as a consequence. Type 3 ulcers are positioned close to the pylorus and are also associated with excessive acid secretion with haemorrhage and perforation also being more common. Type 4 ulcers are rarer and situated close to the gastro–oesophageal junction; they are associated with hypochloryhdria, perforation and elevated operative mortality. Type 5 ulcers may be situated anywhere in the stomach and are associated with chronic NSAID and aspirin use. Important risk factors that precipitate this condition include NSAIDs, which inhibit prostaglandins, leading to a reduced mucosal barrier, alcohol, steroid ingestion, acute stress and major operations. A Cushing's ulcer arises following head injury, whilst Curling's ulcer is due to severe burns.

Important features in the history include epigastric tenderness, which is related to food ingestion and often nocturnal. Duodenal ulcers are more common and often relieved by eating and drinking milk, conversely gastric ulcer pain is precipitated by eating. Anecdotally, patients often point to a singular source of dull, gnawing pain known as the 'pointing sign'. Other important features to note include early satiety, nausea and vomiting (pyloric stenosis), succussion splash (gastric outlet obstruction), diarrhoea (Zollinger–Ellison syndrome) and signs of anaemia and shock (GI bleeding).

Important investigations include FBC to look for active anaemia, *H. pylori* breath/stool tests, stool haem investigations and lastly upper GI endoscopy. If Zollinger–Ellison syndrome is suspected, fasting serum gastrin levels should be considered. In a non-actively bleeding ulcer, *H. pylori*-positive patients should undergo eradication therapy. This can be a number of regimes, examples follow (this may differ from trust to trust):

Triple therapy: PPI, clarithromycin and (amoxicillin or metronidazole);

Sequential therapy: PPI, amoxicillin, clarithromycin and tinidazole; and

Quadruple therapy: PPI, bismuth, metronidazole and tetracycline.

If *H. pylori* is negative, one should treat the underlying cause, such as stopping NSAIDs combined with ulcer healing therapy which includes a PPI as a first line treatment, H2 receptor antagonists or sucralfate or misoprostol as a second line treatment.

In actively bleeding ulcers, risk factors such as NSAIDs and aspirin should be stopped and the patient should receive endoscopy to treat the ulcer. Concurrent use of a PPI has been shown to reduce rebleeding rates and repeat surgery, though there is no effect on mortality. Finally, surgical management is reserved for patients with perforated ulcers, or when endoscopic intervention fails. This decision can also be guided by factors that influence operative mortality and include age, length of time from perforation to admission, co-morbidities and the presence of shock on admission. Postoperatively, the *H. pylori* status of the patient should be checked.

Clinical vignettes for further practice

A 45-year-old male presents with sudden gnawing pain in the epigastric region. He works as a truck driver and has not eaten since the morning as he was running late for work. He has vomited once and described large dark masses in the vomitus. He has no significant past medical history, admits to heavy smoking and drinks moderately every week. He appears pale and clammy and his observations are:

Blood pressure: 133/79 mmHg; HR: 122; RR: 22; Oxygen sats: 97%.

> *Although very tedious, practise different versions of a given surgical topic. As I went through different patient scenarios, I found that my answers became more natural and less robotic. It also forced me to think about the questions I was being asked instead of just regurgitating answers I had memorised.*

2.4 ACUTE ABDOMEN III

Clinical Case

A 23-year-old male presents to A/E with a 2-day history of right-sided abdominal pain. He described the discomfort as a stabbing pain that is constant, started suddenly and has gradually worsened with radiation to his back. He has felt nauseated and vomited multiple times. He denies any preceeding diarrhoea, travel history or eating any take-away food. He mentions no other relevant history, is opening his bowels and is otherwise fit and well. On examination his abdomen is soft, tender in the right upper quadrant with a positive Murphy's sign. All other systems are normal.

HR: 85; BP: 125/80 mmHg; RR: 16; Sats: 99% on air; Temp: 38.1

'How would you proceed with this patient?'

I would resuscitate the patient and assess their level of health using the ALS protocol A, B, C. Starting with airway I would speak with the patient and ensure there was a patent airway and no escalation was needed. I would briefly examine the chest for any gross pathologies based on inspection, palpation, percussion and auscultation of lung fields. At circulation I would asses the fluids status of the patient by examining the skin turgor, capillary refill, tongue hydration, JVP and signs of peripheral oedema. I would gain intravenous access and review adjuncts such as the oxygen saturation, ECG monitoring and blood pressure monitoring. I would react to any abnormal clinical findings and initiate therapy at which point I would reassess the patient. Once the patient is stable I would then take a focused history based on the patient's presenting complaint and relevant past medical, drug and social history.

'What are your differentials and primary diagnosis?'

My primary diagnosis in this patient would be acute cholecystitis supported by the history of right upper quadrant pain, nausea, vomiting and fever. On examination the pain appears typical with a positive Murphy's sign. My differentials would include pancreatitis which may be a complication of the patient having cholecystitis. Although not jaundiced and not presenting with rigors this patient may also have an acute cholangitis. Other less likely differentials include peptic ulcer disease.

'What investigations would you perform?'

After stabilising the patient I would request a urine dipstick to ensure there was no urinary tract infection. Since the patient has signs of sepsis evidenced by fever this would also be part of a septic screen. I would take bloods particularly an FBC to look for a raised WCC and neutrophils, CRP for signs of inflammation, urea and electrolytes which would be more helpful as a baseline should the patient require investigations that involve contrast medium. LFTs would be very important, particularly signs of elevated ALP, GGT and bilirubin, which would support a cholestatic picture. Amylase would also be important to exclude a viable differential in this patient who has features in this history of pancreatitis. I would move on to an erect CXR to exclude a perforated viscus and finally request an ultrasound scan of the abdomen to look for signs of a thickened gallbladder, calculi and pericholecystic fluid. A sonographic Murphy's sign would also support my primary diagnosis. I would be less inclined to do an abdominal film since there is no sign of obstruction and the investigation would be less helpful.

'The following blood test results arrive. How would you interpret these?'

Hb:	14.6
WCC:	13.5
Neutrophils:	8.4

Sodium:	139
Potassium:	3.8
Urea:	4.5
Creatinine:	71
Albumin:	42
Bilirubin:	10
ALT:	50
ALP:	62
GGT:	214

Glucose:	8.5	**ABG:** (On air)	
Amylase:	2645	pH: 7.39	
CRP:	<4	PaO_2: 12.1	
		$PaCO_2$: 5.62	
		Lactate: 2.0	

The blood results appear to show grossly normal hepatic and renal results however there are signs of infection with raised WCC and neutrophils and importantly a significantly raised amylase. The ABG is also grossly normal with all figures in normal parameters. This patient may be suffering from pancreatitis due to gallstones. The gallbladder may or may not be inflammed representing 2 potential pathologies.

'What are the diagnostic criteria for acute cholecystitis?'

To confirm cholecystitis I would examine local signs, systemic signs and radiological signs. Local indicators would include signs of inflammation as evidenced by right upper quadrant pain, tenderness and possibly a palpable mass. I would expect a positive Murphy's sign. Systemically the patient may have a fever, elevated WCC, neutrophils and CRP. Finally radiological signs may show a thickened gallbladder, calculi or a positive sonographic Murphy's sign.

'The US scan report is below. The consultant does not wish for operative management at the moment. How would you manage this patient?'

'Gallbladder demonstrates a significantly thickened and oedematous wall, no stones are present within the gallbladder, there is a small amount of biliary sludge. The common bile duct is of a normal calibre.'

As my senior has already advised against an operative plan I would initiate supportive therapy for this patient. I would place the patient nil by mouth initially in order to rest the gut and pancreas with concomitant IV fluids and IV antibiotics according to local protocol. I would ensure the patient had adequate analgesic preferably with NSAIDS due to their inhibition of prostaglandin and their effects on the gallbladder. I would ensure the patient received gastric protection with a proton pump inhibitor. Alongside this treatment I would ensure close monitoring of adjuncts such as blood pressure, ECG, oxygen saturations and pulse rate. For pancreatitis I would then score the patient according to the Ranson criteria and assess the patient's condition regularly for signs of improvement following therapy.

Background Information

Acute cholecystitis results from acute gallbladder inflammation most often due to the impaction of gallstones at various anatomical sites in the biliary tree including the gallbladder itself, cystic duct or common bile duct.

Patients typically present with intense right upper quadrant pain which although described as biliary colic in many textbooks tends to plateau and be constant. Patients will often describe consuming a fatty meal with pain following shortly afterwards. Associated features include nausea, vomiting and loss of appetite. Prolonged inflammation can cause complications such as abscess or perforation which may manifest as fever. Jaundice can occur in a minority of patients secondary to inflammatory impact upon the biliary tract or calculi causing obstruction in the common bile duct. On examination Murphy's sign describes pain on palpation of the right upper quadrant on deep inspiration. This is of such severity that the patient cannot complete a full inspiration. When elicited using an ultrasound scanner this is described as a sonographic Murphy's sign. A segment of patients may also present with a palpable mass in the right upper quadrant representing a distended gallbladder. Diaphragmatic irritation from an inflamed gallbladder can manifest as right shoulder tip pain.

Other investigations to consider include an abdominal radiograph which can show gallstones and gas in the gallbladder or biliary tree in severe disease. A CT scan of the abdomen is less helpful than an US scan but can demonstrate gallbladder inflammation and other differentials. An MRI scan of the abdomen is helpful in pregnant patients where a CT scan is not appropriate and views can be difficult on US scan. Cholescintigraphy involves the injection of dye that reveals gallbladder filling defects, helpful if after US scan the diagnosis is still unclear.

Indications for abdominal radiographs from the Royal College of Radiologists guidelines:

Indicated

- Perforation
- Obstruction
- Acute inflammatory bowel disease
- Haematuria
- Renal calculi

Not indicated

- Acute GI bleed
- Haematemesis
- Constipation
- Gallstones
- Pancreatitis
- UTI
- Renal/Colonic masses

Sonographic criteria for acute cholecystitis include:

- Distended and thickened gallbladder (>4mm)
- Presence of gallstones
- Pericholecystic fluid
- Positive sonographic Murphy's sign (specificity >90%)

Although still an area of debate regarding operative management of cholecystitis, early laparoscopic cholecystectomy is still recommended as the optimal treatment in mild disease within 72 hours of symptom onset. This also applies to patients suffering from pancreatitis secondary to gallstones. Delaying operative treatment has shown recurrence and need for intervention before patients undergo an elective operative. Early treatment is also superior due to reduced hospital stays though there is no reduction in the proportion of patients undergoing conversion to open procedures. A percutaneous cholecystectomy tube can be considered in a patient not for surgery or who are responding poorly to conservative treatment.

Clinical vignettes for further practice

A 28-year-old female presents with a 3-hour history of severe right upper quadrant pain, nausea and vomiting. The pain started shortly after eating a fatty take-away meal. She denies any diarrhoea and her friends who ate the same food are well. She is otherwise fit and healthy. On examination her observations are within normal limits except for a mild tachycardia and pain in the right upper quadrant with shoulder tip pain.

> I was definitely unprepared for my clinical station vignette and the questioning during the interview. I had looked over topics and did questions as part of my revision. I prepared from flash cards and thought I had a good knowledge base around the common surgical presentations. During the station it becomes very clear theoretical knowledge is far less useful than clinical experience and interview practice. My mind went completely blank on topics that I had practised and memorised. If I could have the time back I would have spent much more time practising scenario questions and being placed under pressure.

2.5 ANORECTAL DISEASE

Clinical case

As the surgical SHO on-call you are referred a 39-year-old male who complains of a 2-week history of extreme perianal pain. The patient described exquisite pain when opening their bowels and has become distressed at the sight of fresh blood noticed on wiping and occasionally in the pan. The pain typically lasts for 10–15 minutes after defaecation. The patient has avoided eating for the last few days to try to avoid the pain. The patient denies suffering fever, urinary symptoms, episodes of diarrhoea or any other abnormality. They are otherwise fit and healthy. Basic observations are all within normal range.

'What is your primary, single diagnosis for this patient?'

I believe this patient is suffering from an acute anal fissure.

'How would you proceed with this patient?'

I would begin by formally resuscitating the patient myself and assess their level of health using the ALS protocol A, B, C. Once the patient is stable, I would take a formal history to confirm the details of the referral and to reiterate any formal colorectal-based investigations. Among other facts, I would enquire in more depth about the diet of the patient, episodes of straining, the quantity and nature of the bleeding in terms of volume and if there were any clots. I would also identify any measures the patient had taken including pharmaceutical aids such as laxatives to help with their symptoms. I would take the opportunity to examine the patient, particularly the abdominal system, after offering a chaperone I would with extreme care attempt a PR examination.

> Although it can be exhausting during your interview practice, do not ever omit your resuscitation of the patient. This demonstrates your approach to safe clinical practice. Although tedious, you should create a common statement at the start of your answers, when appropriate, to safely resuscitate your patients. This should be mandatory as you otherwise risk failing the station entirely.

'Why would you perform a PR examination when it is likely to cause pain to the patient with an anal fissure?'

At all times, I would ensure that I was being compassionate and considerate to the patient and avoid all actions not in the best interest of the patient. However, at least attempting a PR examination is indicated as the associated discomfort is characteristic and supportive towards a diagnosis of an anal fissure. Also, the PR examination helps to exclude my differential diagnoses which can present similarly such as strangulated or thrombosed piles.

'Upon examination, how would you differentiate between your alternative diagnoses?'

My differentials would include anal fissure, haemorrhoids and anal fistula. On examination for an anal fissure, I would first expect the examination to be too painful for the patient and the area of interest would often be concealed due to anal spasm even with analgesic aids. At this juncture, I would not proceed with the examination and consider an examination under anaesthesia. If I was able to examine the anorectal area, I would expect to see a superficial tear in the anoderm and possibly white circular fibres which represent the internal sphincter. Although this is most likely an acute fissure, in chronic disease a sentinel tag is often present. For haemorrhoids on inspection I would expect to see masses with a blue or purple discolouration at the anus. Upon palpation, they are usually painless and soft masses but can be inflamed, painful and engorged. Finally, for an anal fistula there may be purulent discharge, surrounding erythema and also a fluctuant indurated mass. Although difficult for the patient there can occasionally be soiling of the undergarments due to discharge, and I would consider examining these also.

'Describe the different classes of haemorrhoids.'

There are four classifications or grades of haemorrhoids. In grade 1, the protrusions are limited to within the anal canal, and they tend to present as painless bleeding. In grade 2, the haemorrhoids protrude beyond the anal canal but reduce spontaneously; they are associated with mild pain, bleeding and pruritus. Grade 3 haemorrhoids can involve painful bleeding and require manual reduction. Grade 4 haemorrhoids are the most severe, being irreducible and often associated with discharge, ulcers and fluctuant masses.

'What treatment would you offer this patient with an uncomplicated fissure?'

I would first ensure that the patient was made comfortable with appropriate analgesic. Following this, I would offer conservative treatment first which would include a high fibre diet and elevated fluid intake. I would recommend sitz baths as well as stool softeners. For topical analgesic, I would offer GTN but avoid it for pregnant or lactating patients. I would warn the patient about headaches with this therapy and recommend paracetamol which is often helpful. Diltiazem is an alternative if headaches do not abate.

'What treatment would you offer a patient with resistant anal fissures?'

If conservative measures failed, I would then consider more invasive measures beginning with botulinum toxin. In more severe disease, a sphincterotomy can be performed but I would warn the patient of the risk of incontinence. Alternatives to this option include an anal advancement flap.

Background information

Anal fissures are longitudinal tears that traverse the skin and mucosa typically in the lower third of the anal canal. Although constipation is commonly believed to precipitate anal fissures, there is no clear evidence towards this and indeed constipation may arise due to anal spasm secondary to an anal fissure. Patients using opiate-based analgesic are shown to have a higher incidence of anal fissures. The underlying pathology involves local trauma, which causes internal and external anal sphincter dysfunction and eventually ischaemia. This is believed to be as valid as the theory that hard stools cause tears in the anal skin. More than 90% of fissures occur in the posterior midline, anterior fissures tend to occur in women especially following childbirth. Anal fissures are the most commonly associated anal abnormality in Crohn's disease. Alongside anal pain, patients may also present with bright red bleeding, pruritus ani, watery discharge and constipation.

Fissures may be classified as acute or chronic. Most acute fissures tend to heal over 1–2 weeks while chronic fissures persist for more than 6 weeks. Accompanying features in the latter include visible sphincter fibres, indurated skin edges and a sentinel skin tag. Important differentials to consider in patients with anal pain include:

- Perianal haematoma
- Perianal abscess
- Inflammatory bowel disease
- Strangulated internal haemorrhoids
- Proctalgia fugax
- Colorectal carcinoma

Clinical vignettes for further practice

1. A 35-year-old female presents with severe pain when opening her bowels for the last 2 months. This is associated with intense itching in the area and frank bleeding. She has noticed cycles of recovery and then a return of her symptoms.

2. A 44-year-old male presents with a 4-day history of painless bleeding per recta. The blood is bright red and often mixed with the stool or present on wiping. The patient admits to a mostly fast-food and take-away diet, and has a visibly large body habitus.

" *My clinical station initially went really well. The vignette covered a topic that I had revised well and practised. As soon as the interview started, I was able to answer questions confidently until I mentioned my differentials. The entire conversation then shifted and we were talking about an entirely different topic. I don't know if they felt I was competent in the vignette topic, but I felt completely derailed with the new line of questioning. It's difficult to switch your mind from focusing on one topic to a different one, and wasn't something I had thought about beforehand.* "

2.6 BACK PAIN

Clinical case

You are asked to see a 62-year-old female who has presented to A/E with an acute onset of lower back pain. The pain started suddenly 12 hours ago and has been increasing in intensity. The patient was shopping when the pain initially started, and it is gnawing in nature. The patient is unable to get comfortable in any position and also cannot identify a particular precipitating factor, such as movement. She suffers from hypertension only and, although on medication, has not been reviewed in years. She admits to moderate social alcohol intake.

'How would you proceed with this patient?'

I would resuscitate the patient and assess their level of health using the ALS protocol A, B, C and also ask for senior and nursing assistance. Starting with the airway, I would speak with the patient and ensure there was a patent airway and no escalation was needed. I would initiate high-flow oxygen through a non-rebreather mask, adjusting this decision if needed later. I would briefly examine the chest for gross pathologies. At circulation, I would ensure there were two large bore grey cannulae placed at both antecubital fossae, oxygen saturation, ECG monitoring and blood pressure monitoring.

I would request a full set of bloods for any pathology including FBC, U&E, LFTs, clotting and crossmatch for 4 units of blood. I would also order an ABG to review acid-base status, oxygenation and lactate levels. I would examine the patient's cardiovascular system and assess their haemodynamic status based on capillary refill, presence of pallor, pulse rate, rhythm and nature and praecordium examination findings. I would react to any abnormal clinical findings and initiate therapy, after which I would reassess the patient.

> Presenting candidates with a sick patient is the easiest way to determine who are the best prepared and most competent. Completing ALS and ATLS courses are extremely helpful in this regard. Nevertheless, you should still practise your resuscitation routine with as many variations and questions as possible.

'Assuming the patient is stable after resuscitation, what would you do next?'

I would take a focused history to clarify and confirm the referral details. In addition, I would ask for specific details pertinent to my primary suspicion of aortic aneurysm. I would ascertain for any past medical or family history of connective tissue disorders, hyperlipidaemia and COPD and determine if the patient is a smoker. I would specifically like to examine the patient's abdomen for an expansile, pulsatile mass above the umbilicus. If I discovered this, I would request for immediate escalation to a senior. I would also examine the popliteal and femoral vessels for signs of aneurysm.

'What investigations would you consider if your examination findings were positive?'

I would ideally request an abdominal ultrasound scan to confirm my suspicions and also document the size of the aneurysm. An abdominal FAST ultrasound scan can be performed in A/E, if appropriate. Other investigations that may be appropriate include a CT scan with contrast if the patient's renal function permits, an MRI scan or an MR angiography.

'What are your other differentials for this patient?'

Differential	Symptoms/signs	Investigations
Diverticulitis	Often localises to the left quadrant occasionally with abdominal fullness. There is no pulsatile abdominal mass	Positive stool guaiac test Leukocytosis CT scan may show diverticulae and its related sequelae
Renal colic	Pain is typically from loin to groin. May be associated with nausea, vomiting and haematuria	Urine analysis may show haematuria with/without infection. US or CT KUB may confirm renal stones
Inflammatory bowel disease	Crampy abdominal pain, which is often left-sided. Abdominal examination may yield abdominal masses	FBC often shows anaemia. Endoscopy usually confirms IBD findings
Appendicitis	Central pain that typically migrates to the right iliac fossa. A mass may be palpable in the right iliac fossa	Bloods may show a leukocytosis and raised inflammatory markers. An US or CT usually confirms an inflamed appendix
GI haemorrhage	History and examination may mimic an aortic rupture	Positive stool guaiac test. Endoscopy confirms bleeding source

Following resuscitation, a nurse informs you of the following observations for the patient:

HR: 120; RR: 30; BP: 88/59 mmHg and Sats: 92% on air.

'Describe the level of shock for this patient.'

This patient is suffering from a class III shock based on the low blood pressure, which is a late sign of shock alongside a tachycardia of 120 bpm. I would additionally support this by speaking to the patient and ascertaining her level of consciousness and measuring her urine output. I would address these results by again escalating as a matter of urgency to a senior surgical team member that the patient may have suffered a ruptured aortic aneurysm. I would then begin fluid resuscitation with crystalloids and blood once available. If I was in a centre equipped for suitable vascular surgery, I would also begin preparation for potential operative management prophylactically by alerting the nursing staff, placing the patient nil by mouth and alerting the theatre staff and anaesthetist. I would ensure that a member of the patient's family was alerted to the situation.

	Class I	Class II	Class III	Class IV
Blood loss (mL)	≤750	750–1500	1500–2000	>2000
Blood loss (%)	0–15	15–30	30–40	>40
Heart rate	<100	>100	>120	>140
Blood pressure	Normal	Normal	Decreased	Decreased
Pulse pressure	Normal	Decreased	Decreased	Decreased
Respiratory rate	14–20	20–30	30–40	>35
Urine output (mL/H)	>30	20–30	5–15	Minimal
Mental status	Normal	Anxious	Confused	Confused and lethargic
Fluid replacement	Crystalloid	Crystalloid	Crystalloid and blood	Crystalloid and blood

'Briefly describe the supportive management of a ruptured abdominal aortic aneurysm (AAA).'

I would be vigilant for a patient with a ruptured aortic aneurysm, who often presents with a triad of hypotension, an expansile pulsatile mass and pain, which is usually abdominal or back pain. Supportive resuscitation involves oxygenation via adjuncts or intubation, and insertion of a central venous, urinary and arterial catheter. Finally, I would establish close communications with the anaesthetist, intensive care and theatre departments. I would be cautious with my level of fluid resuscitation in a patient with known rupture, and follow the principle of hypotensive resuscitation which prevents dilutional coagulopathy and a secondary clot from being disrupted due to aggressive fluid infusion. I would therefore aim for a systolic blood pressure of no greater than 50–70 mm Hg, under the strict guidance of a senior anaesthetist and consultant surgeons.

'What operative management would you expect in this patient?'

For this patient, the management may be via an endovascular aneurysm repair, otherwise known as EVAR, which is known to be the most effective repair; however, this is dependent upon the aortoiliac anatomy, which is not available in this patient. If an EVAR procedure cannot be performed then an open aneurysm repair can be attempted. Unfortunately, most patients who suffer an aneurysm do not reach the operating room. The mortality for those patients who are operated on is 50%.

'What conservative measures would you advise for a patient with an incidental small AAA?'

My management for a patient with this pathology would centre around surveillance, control of risk factors and treatment of cardiovascular disease. For infra-renal AAA's, 6–12 month ultrasound or CT scanning should be undertaken while aneurysms <4.0 cm can be reviewed every 2–3 years. With regards to risk factors I would encourage a healthier diet and smoking cessation. Finally, I would aggressively treat any identified cardiovascular disease such as hypertension.

Background information

Although the consequences of an abdominal aortic aneurysm are catastrophic, the majority of aneurysms are asymptomatic and discovered incidentally. Abdominal and back pain are the most common symptomatic presentations. An aneurysm is commonly defined as a pathological dilatation more than 1.5 cm of its natural diameter. The average diameter is 3 cm and the vast majority of aneurysms that are infra-renal. Important risk factors include cigarette smoking, family history of aneurysms, increasing age and congenital or connective tissue disease. Interestingly, male sex is a predisposing factor for prevalence, while female sex is more commonly associated with rupture. Aneurysm palpation is found to be accurate only in patients with a lean body habitus and a diameter >5 cm. The causes are considered multifactorial though the underlying pathophysiology remains consistent with aortic elastic medial degeneration and cystic medial necrosis.

Screening guidelines are important, and you should be well versed in the following recommendations:

1. Patients aged ≥65 years may undergo a single ultrasound session for discovery of incidental disease;
2. If the aneurysm is <3 cm wide, no further follow-up is recommended;
3. If the aneurysm is 3.0–4.4 cm, a repeat of US scans in 12 months is recommended;
4. If the aneurysm is 4.5–5.4 cm^3, monthly US scans are recommended; and
5. If the aneurysm is 5.5 cm or more, a specialist review is recommended.

Selected investigations to consider include:

Investigation	Justification
FBC	Signs of anaemia which may indicate a patient in shock Leukocytosis which may support an infective aneurysm
ESR/CRP	Elevation may support an inflammatory aneurysm
Blood cultures	Appropriate if an infective aneurysm is suspected
US	Definitive investigation for diagnosis of aneurysm
CT	Helpful for intra-luminal pathology, also helpful if the origin is close or proximal to the renal arteries
MRI	If contrast use is not compatible, e.g. allergy
Aortography	Helpful in documenting occlusive disease, and also in patients unable to undergo CT scanning

Treatment

- **Ruptured AAA:** EVAR is the first-choice intervention; if complicated by aorto-iliac disease, open repair is performed. Broad-spectrum perioperative antibiotic cover is also indicated.
- **Symptomatic patient without rupture:** EVAR is the first-choice intervention; if complicated by aorto-iliac disease, open repair is performed. Administer preoperative beta blockers and co-morbidity treatment.

Clinical vignettes for further practice

1. A 68-year-old male is invited for a general health screen. He is on treatment for hyperlipidaemia which is well controlled, but is otherwise in good health. On examination a palpable, expansile mass is discovered.

2. A 52-year-old male presents to A/E with a 1-day history of increasing sharp pain in the centre of the abdomen. He suffers from diabetes, hypertension and smokes 10 cigarettes a day. He is clinically stable but despite analgesic remains in pain. An US scan in A/E shows a 5.2 cm aneurysm.

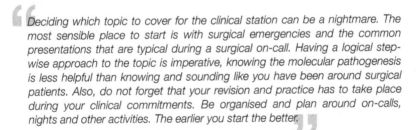

Deciding which topic to cover for the clinical station can be a nightmare. The most sensible place to start is with surgical emergencies and the common presentations that are typical during a surgical on-call. Having a logical step-wise approach to the topic is imperative, knowing the molecular pathogenesis is less helpful than knowing and sounding like you have been around surgical patients. Also, do not forget that your revision and practice has to take place during your clinical commitments. Be organised and plan around on-calls, nights and other activities. The earlier you start the better.

2.7 BOWEL OBSTRUCTION I

Clinical case

Whilst on the surgical ward, an FY1 doctor asks your advice about a postoperative patient. They present a 49-year-old male who underwent an extended right hemicolectomy for colorectal carcinoma two days ago. The operative note details no complications and instructs opiate-based analgesic and clear fluids in the postoperative period. The patient was comfortable yesterday, but today complains of abdominal pain and nausea. The nursing staff have noted multiple episodes of vomiting. Upon examination, the junior doctor reports a distended abdomen with absent bowel sounds. PR examination reveals an empty rectum. The wound site appears clean and unremarkable.

'What causes of mechanical bowel obstruction do you know?'

Bowel obstruction may be mechanical or non-mechanical and often presents with similar symptoms and signs. Causes of mechanical bowel obstruction may be classed as intra-luminal, mural and extra-mural. Intra-luminal causes include faecal impaction, food bolus, foreign bodies, intussusception (in children) and rarely gallstones causing ileus. Mural causes include inflammatory bowel disease, diverticular disease and carcinoma. Extra-mural causes include volvulus, strangulated hernias and adhesions.

> Receiving a handover from a colleague is an important yet precarious situation. You must convey to the interviewer your respect for your colleague when they ask your advice and appreciate any urgency in their referral. You must also confirm the referral details yourself once the patient is stable.

'What specific features would you be interested in concerning the history of this patient for bowel obstruction?'

I would begin by formally resuscitating the patient myself and assessing their level of health using the ALS protocol A, B, C. Once the patient is stable, I would then wish to clarify the junior doctor's history, and confirm the examination findings. The important symptoms and signs of bowel obstruction I would identify include colicky abdominal pain, distension, constipation and vomiting. I would first consider the risk factors important in this patient such as recent abdominal surgery, medical conditions such as pneumonia and pancreatitis. Increasing analgesic use to control pain would also be important. I would also identify more systemic problems such as sepsis. With regards to the history, I would clarify the patient's degree of nausea and vomiting episodes, as these may be an indication for nasogastric tube insertion. I would characterise the patient's abdominal pain, cramping and discomfort as typical in

> Keeping a structure to your answers will help you to remember various causes or pathologies. It is also easier for the interviewer to follow a packaged answer that is organised rather than a long list in a random order.

mechanical obstruction whilst in ileus they are less obvious. Finally, I would document the passage of flatus and stool from the patient and whether there was any absolute constipation.

'What specific features would you be interested in upon the examination of this patient for bowel obstruction?'

On inspection, I would look for abdominal distension though this is not specific for the pathology. I would also look for causes of obstruction such as hernias. During palpation, I would try to elicit evidence of peritoneal inflammation such as rigidity, rebound tenderness and guarding. Percussion may reveal tympanic sounds in keeping with flatus or gas trapped in the abdominal cavity. More dull sounds may support faecal matter. Upon auscultation, hyperactive sounds may support small bowel obstruction whilst absent bowel sounds would be more in keeping with an ileus, though this is again non-specific. Finally, a PR examination would be helpful to look for impacted faecal matter.

'Present this abdominal radiograph.'

'This is an abdominal radiograph without any clinical identifiers including patient details, time and date of imaging. There are visible dilated loops of bowel around the centre of the abdomen with valvulae conniventes present. There does not appear to be any faecal loading, or any other signs of pathology. The bone architecture appears normal with no obvious visceral anomalies. This is in keeping with a small bowel obstruction. I would also consider an erect CXR, imaging of the abdomen after injection of water-soluble contrast through a nasogastric tube, an abdominal ultrasound or CT scan.'

The radiograph shows minimal distension of several small bowel loops suspicious of obstruction. The small bowel would usually be centrally located and would have valvulae conniventes. The maximum normal diameter of the small bowel is 3 cm. An erect abdominal film may also show multiple fluid levels, demonstrating a 'ladder' pattern.

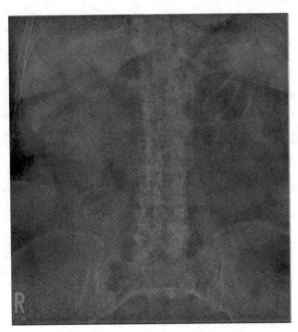

'How would you manage the fluid resuscitation of the patient?'

I would resuscitate the patient and assess their level of health using the ALS protocol A, B, C. Once stable, I would place the patient nil by mouth, consider the insertion of a nasogastric tube and gain intravenous access for fluid resuscitation. I would assess the patient's co-morbidity status such as heart failure, as well as hydration status by examining the mucosal membranes, skin turgor, pallor, capillary refill, JVP and lung bases. In hypovolaemia, I would consider prescribing a bolus of normal saline or Hartmann's solution. For maintenance, I would assess the patient's fluid and electrolyte requirements in accordance with their co-morbidity and prescribe an appropriate fluid regimen. This may include Hartmann's solution or normal saline in conjunction with 5% dextrose and potassium supplementation.

'You review the patient after 3 days and they are still nil by mouth and on fluid resuscitation. How would you proceed?'

Although not ideal, patients suffering from an ileus may need to be kept nil by mouth with intravenous supplementation for a prolonged period of time. When this period begins to exceed 7 days, the benefits of parenteral nutrition begin to outweigh the risks. I would liase with the senior members of the team, a dietician and the patient to facilitate this while the bowel is allowed to rest. I would also ensure that regular electrolyte checks are performed.

Background information

An ileus can be described as a reduction in gastrointestinal motility not caused by mechanical obstruction. It commonly follows operative management involving laparotomy rather than laparoscopy, and can typically last 48–72 hours, however in many cases this period can be significantly prolonged. Treatment is centred around keeping patients nil by mouth in order to rest the gut, allow for the identification of precipitating factors and continue supportive therapy. Iatrogenic factors are a common culprit and often replacing opiate-based analgesic with NSAIDs helps to prevent a worsening ileus. Other treatment options include early enteral feeding and ambulation. Other important causative factors to consider include:

- Electrolyte disturbances
- Inflammatory responses
- Iatrogenic compounds such as analgesic, anticholinergics and anaesthesia
- Acute or systemic disease, e.g. acute cholecystitis, myocardial infarction pancreatitis and sepsis
- Multi-organ trauma

Clinical vignettes for further practice

A 66-year-old female presents with postoperative intermittent abdominal pain, nausea and vomiting 8 days after her initial operation. She complains of vague abdominal discomfort and bloating following a laparotomy for a suspected bowel perforation. She is nil by mouth at present and on intravenous fluid therapy.

> *I practised for the interviews mostly by revising general surgery topics and reviewing my notes from MRCS and surgical finals at medschool. I didn't get through first time round. The second time I was successful because I completely changed my method. I focused more on scenarios and then read around topics later. Work through a patient from presentation, diagnosis, investigations, etc. Look at investigations such as x-rays, CT scans, etc. Although images didn't come up in my interview, questions about investigations and what I would look for came up both times.*

2.8 BOWEL OBSTRUCTION II

Clinical case

You are referred a patient during a night on-call. The A/E team present a 69-year-old male with acute colicky abdominal pain. He has been feeling nauseated and vomited in the A/E. He has experienced urgency to open his bowel but has been unable to pass flatus or faeces for 12 hours. He admits to some passage of blood mixed in with stool in the last 2 weeks, but was hoping this would pass. He has also noticed significant unintentional weight loss in the last 3 months. You arrive in A/E as the nursing staff record his basic observations:

Heart rate: 95; Blood pressure: 135/80 mmHg; Resp rate: 16; Sats: 99%

'How would you proceed with this patient?'

I would resuscitate the patient and assess his level of health using the ALS protocol A, B, C. Starting with the airway, I would speak with the patient and ensure there was a patent airway and no escalation was needed. I would briefly examine the chest for any gross pathologies based on inspection, palpation, percussion and auscultation of the lung fields. For circulation, I would asses the fluids status of the patient by examining the skin turgor, capillary refill, tongue hydration, JVP and signs of peripheral oedema. I would gain intravenous access and also examine the monitoring adjuncts such as oxygen saturation, ECG monitoring and blood pressure monitoring. I would examine the patient's cardiovascular system including the praecordium. I would react to any abnormal clinical findings and initiate therapy, at which point I would reassess the patient. Once the patient is stable, I would then take a focused history based on the patient's presenting complaint and relevant past medical and drug history and as well social circumstances.

'What investigations would you consider for this patient?'

I would start with a urine analysis to identify signs of urinary infection and renal disease. For bloods, I would request an FBC, U&E, LFTs, amylase, coagulation and CRP. I would also request an ECG and then importantly consider an erect CXR and abdominal film, and discuss with the radiologist if necessary. Depending on the results of these investigations, I would then consider more invasive, specialist investigations.

Investigation	Justification
FBC	Microcytic anaemia may be suggestive of a colorectal malignancy, especially right-sided neoplasms. Raised WCC can indicate peritonitis
U&E	Obstruction can result in electrolyte imbalances particularly hypokalaemia
Renal function	Baseline renal function is important if more invasive investigations are to be considered, as well as indicating the degree of hydration
Amylase	Intra-abdominal pathology can cause elevation. Helpful to consider other causes such as pancreatitis
Coagulation	Coagulopathy can result from sepsis
Erect CXR	Free subdiaphragmatic air can indicate a perforation requiring urgent management. The absence of this sign does not exclude a viscus perforation
AXR	Evidence of dilated loops of bowel can confirm diagnosis. Normal limits include: caecum: 10–12 cm, ascending colon: 8 cm, rectosigmoid area: 6–7 cm

'If an erect CXR showed air under the diaphragm, what would be your differentials?'

My primary differential that I would wish to exclude would be a viscus perforation, such as that resulting from acute appendicitis, diverticulitis, bowel perforation and ruptured peptic ulcer. My other differentials would include recent significant abdominal surgery, such as a laparotomy or prolonged laparoscopic surgery. Other causes include patients suffering from COPD with gas escaping from the tracheobronchial tree. Finally, I would consider the possibility of Chilaiditi's sign, which describes the interposition of the transverse colon between the liver and diaphragm, and hence appears as subphrenic gas.

'Based on this radiograph and assuming the patient is stable, what other investigations would you consider?'

Based on the patient's presenting complaints and the investigation findings so far, this patient appears to be suffering from a form of bowel obstruction. I would therefore alert my senior in surgery and discuss with the radiologist about performing a CT scan of the abdomen. This has excellent accuracy in diagnosing obstructions. The scan may not only confirm an obstruction, but be useful in revealing the underlying cause and other diagnostic parameters. I would ensure the patient's renal function was not deranged, as contrast would be preferable. Other investigations to consider include a contrast study such as water-soluble contrast, and less commonly a barium enema. This can also be helpful in giving the location of the obstruction, its severity and diagnosis, though it is much less accurate than a CT scan. I would not suggest this study in a patient with perforation or peritonitis.

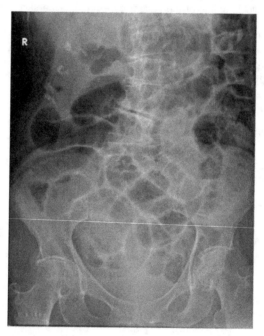

Finally, a flexible or rigid endoscopy is particularly helpful in a volvulus, as it serves both diagnostic and therapeutic purposes. I would not suggest this in a patient at risk of perforation, such as inflammatory bowel disease or diverticulitis.

'The CT scan confirms an obstructing colorectal carcinoma, what general surgical options do you know?'

In this situation, surgical management would aim to relieve the obstruction and where possible resect the offending lesion for analysis. There are various anastomotic and postoperative options. A defunctioning ileostomy or colostomy proximal to the obstruction is helpful, particularly in ill or high-risk patients that would not withstand resection, or where this option is not possible. A patient with a right-sided obstruction, for example, may have a defunctioning ileostomy whilst those with a left-sided lesion would benefit from defunctioning loop transverse colostomy. In healthier patients, or situations where a resection is possible, more invasive options can be considered. A lesion in the right colon may be resected and a primary anastomosis performed without a defunctioning ileostomy. A subtotal colectomy is also helpful depending on the location of lesions.

Background information

Large bowel obstruction is a surgical emergency and you must act quickly and competently to identify those patients who would benefit from operative or non-operative treatment. This requires efficient work up, optimisation of co-morbidities and the activation of appropriate teams to facilitate treatment.

Patients typically present with a large range of symptoms though the cardinal presentation revolves around nausea, vomiting, colicky abdominal pain, abdominal distension and constipation. Typical symptoms and signs include:

- Colicky abdominal pain
- Nausea
- Vomiting
- Abdominal distension
- Tympanic bowel sounds on percussion
- Changes in bowel habit
- Signs of overflow diarrhoea
- Signs of peritonism, e.g. abdominal pain, rigidity, rebound tenderness, etc.
- PR examination confirming empty rectum or hard impacted stools
- Unintentional, significant weight loss
- Bowel sounds suggestive of obstruction
- PR bleeding
- Signs of anaemia, e.g. shortness of breath, pallor and malaise
- Abdominal masses

The majority of colonic obstructions are secondary to colorectal malignancy. Right-sided tumours tend to be sessile and present with symptoms of anaemia due to prolonged PR bleeding. Left-sided tumours tend to be annular and stenosing, and more typically present with obstructive symptoms. A volvulus of the colon is the next most common abnormality, with sigmoid volvulus being more common than caecal. Strictures and hernia represent the majority of other causes of bowel obstruction; other rarer causes include foreign bodies, pelvic abscess and so on.

All patients should receive supportive resuscitation irrespective of cause. This includes:

1. Provide the patient with appropriate analgesic and antiemetics.
2. Place the patient nil by mouth to rest the bowel and relieve future vomiting.
3. Consider insertion of a nasogastric tube to decompress the bowel and relieve future vomiting.
4. Gain intravenous access and begin fluid resuscitation matched to the patient's hydration status.
5. Fluid input and output charts are helpful alongside urinary catheterisation to aid fluid management.
6. Patients who are being prepared for surgery may benefit from prophylactic antibiotics.
7. Conservative treatment must often be trialled for at least 3 days for effect.

Clinical vignettes for further practice

A 60-year-old female presents with increasing abdominal distension and constipation. She has noticed over the last few weeks changes in her bowel habits, ranging from prolonged constipation to diarrhoea. She has on occasion noticed that her stool is dark coloured. Alongside this, she has noticed a loss of appetite, nausea and pain presenting in a diffuse manner across the abdomen. She has a family history of breast and ovarian cancer.

" *Review your notes and scenarios over and over again. When I first started to practise and review potential scenarios, it's soul-crushing and can seem a huge mountain to climb. With time and practice, you will soon fall into a good rhythm of thought and on repeating the scenarios and questions everything falls into place much more easily. Do not leave your practice to just a few weeks before the interview.* "

2.9 BOWEL OBSTRUCTION III

Clinical case

Your colleague hands over a patient he/she has been referred at the end of his/her shift. It is a 35-year-old female who complains of acute colicky abdominal pain, nausea, vomiting and no passage of flatus for the last 12 hours. She is otherwise fit and well with no significant past medical history except for an open appendicectomy performed 12 months ago. On attending A/E, the patient is writhing with pain.

'How would you proceed with this patient?'

I would resuscitate the patient and assess their level of health using the ALS protocol A, B, C. Starting with the airway, I would speak with the patient and ensure there was a patent airway and no escalation was needed. I would briefly examine the chest for any gross pathologies based on inspection, palpation, percussion and auscultation of the lung fields. For circulation, I would assess the fluids status of the patient by examining the skin turgor, capillary refill, tongue hydration, JVP and signs of peripheral oedema. I would gain intravenous access and also examine the monitoring adjuncts, such as oxygen saturation, ECG monitoring and blood pressure monitoring. After checking for drug allergies, I would prescribe analgesic, antiemetics and intravenous fluids. I would examine the patient's cardiovascular system, including praecordium. I would react to any abnormal clinical findings and initiate therapy, at which point I would reassess the patient.

> Respond to every detail within the vignette. It is just as important to state that you would give analgesic to the patient, as well as follow the resuscitation protocol. Be ready to expand on the WHO analgesic ladder. This guide will highlight the pitfalls that will inevitably be missed by relying solely on theory from textbooks.

Once the patient is stable, I would then take a focused history based on the patient's presenting complaint and relevant past medical and drug history as well as social circumstances. I would also perform a more thorough examination, particularly of the abdominal system.

'How would you differentiate between small bowel and large bowel obstruction clinically?'

Although not very specific, clinically I would expect small bowel obstruction for early nausea and early bilious vomiting, since the obstruction is more proximal. I would expect late abdominal distension and late constipation. Theoretically, since a large bowel obstruction is more distal, I would expect later nausea and vomiting and earlier constipation and abdominal distension.

'What are the common causes of small bowel obstruction?'

The most common causes for small bowel obstruction in the United Kingdom include adhesion formation secondary to abdominal surgery. Other causes are hernias such as inguinal, incisional and umbilical among others – especially if they become obstructed, Crohn's disease, small bowel malignancy and appendicitis.

'What conservative treatment would you use for this patient with the following AXR?'

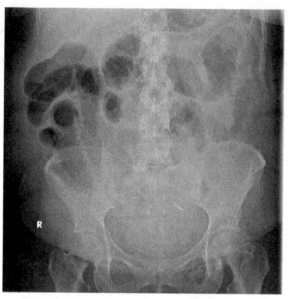

Following resuscitation and appraising the urine dipstick and bloods results, I would then begin my conservative management of this patient. I would place the patient nil by mouth, give appropriate and safe analgesic with antiemetics and also prescribe intravenous fluids. The fluids would aim to initially meet losses and then provide maintenance. I would monitor my therapy by inserting a urinary catheter with an input and output fluid chart. Finally, I would alert my senior to ensure that common treatable causes for small bowel obstruction had not been missed. Also, they can advise if more advanced management is needed, such as an appendicectomy or hernia repair.

I would review the patient regularly over the next 3 days to ensure she is not worsening and for signs of improvement. I would ensure that on day 3 of her review, if there was no improvement and as advised by the consultant, preparations were made for operative management. This may typically involve an exploratory laparotomy, for which I would review worsening serum markers of infection and inflammation, air-fluid levels on abdominal films and persistent or worsening clinical signs of obstruction.

Background information

Small bowel obstruction arises from the compromise of the bowel lumen, resulting in characteristic nausea, vomiting, abdominal pain and constipation. Synonymous with large bowel obstruction, it is considered a surgical emergency requiring meticulous clerking, investigations and management with appropriate escalation.

Small bowel obstruction can be classified in the following manner:

- **Incomplete bowel obstruction:** This usually represents a temporary, reversible intestinal obstruction which responds to conservative treatment. The patient tends to have sporadic bowel movements and passage of flatus, which is usually due to uncomplicated adhesions, hernias and Crohn's disease. Small bowel follow-through investigations will reveal partial passage of the reagent used, and its appearance within the rectum.

- **Complete bowel obstruction:** A complete obstruction of the small bowel is a surgical emergency, which typically involves unwell patients with signs of complete constipation, significant abdominal distension and signs of peritonism. Most patients will require experienced operative intervention as soon as possible since prolonged obstruction can lead to ischaemia, necrosis, perforation and peritonitis, which is fatal in the majority of patients. Small bowel follow-through investigations will reveal no passage beyond the obstruction.

Clinical vignettes for further practice

A 39-year-old obese female patient presents to A/E with an acute central abdominal pain, nausea, vomiting and abdominal distension. She has been recovering from severe acute cholecystitis, for which she is awaiting an elective appointment for laparoscopic cholecystectomy. Upon examination, she looks unwell, her abdomen is soft but markedly distended and PR examination is empty. Abdominal radiographs show multiple air fluid levels.

> " I was asked to state what features I would look for in some of the investigations I mentioned in my answers. When there is an image in front of you, it helps to prompt your mind to mention specific features that are important. It's very helpful to practise analysing investigations because, if challenged, it can be impressive to reel off a list or expand further into the discussion. "

2.10 BREAST DISEASE

Clinical case

You are the surgical CT1 on call and you are referred a 29-year-old female presenting with pains in her left breast. She noticed a lump around her left nipple. After a few days, she became worried as the lump grew in size and became considerably more painful. She denies any discharge from the nipple, weight loss or any other related symptoms. She has recently given birth without complication, and is otherwise fit and well. Upon examination, there is a 2 by 3 cm tender, erythematous mass that is fluctuant on palpation in the peri-areolar region of the upper outer quadrant of the left breast.

'What are your differentials for this patient?'

My primary differential for this patient is a breast abscess which may be secondary to lactation. My secondary differential would be breast malignancy. This can also present as a variably shaped breast mass(es), nipple discharge, surrounding skin oedema or peau d'orange and lymphadenopathy. This could also be a fibrocystic disease, which can present with non-bloody discharge – though I would expect a cyclical history of mastalgia that is related to the menstrual cycle. The patient may also have a milk retention cyst, or galactocele, which can similarly present as a tender lump but is not usually associated with localised breast inflammation or systemic illness.

'What other features would you elicit from the patient regarding their presentation?'

I would ask the patient about a preceeding illness, such as general malaise and flu-like illness, which can be suggestive of mastitis. I would also ask if they had noticed a fever alongside the breast pain, discharge and other masses suggestive of an abscess. Finally, I would elicit risk factors that may predispose to mastitis or the formation of an abscess. This would include poor breast-feeding techniques, poor breast hygiene, aseptic nipple piercings, shaving around the nipple area, recent lactation and infants <2 months old. Previous episodes of mastitis, breast abscesses and nipple injuries would also be important.

'What other breast examination findings would you look for in this patient?'

On gaining the patient's consent for examination, and with the presence of a chaperone, I would examine each of the 4 quadrants of both breasts. I would specifically be looking for signs of nipple discharge, inversion, induration or retraction. For any masses that were present, I would continue to examine for pain, size, shape, texture and fluctuance alongside associated lymphadenopathy.

'What diagnostic investigations or procedures would you consider?'

I would request an FBC and inflammatory markers to primarily examine for underlying infections. If the patient had septic features, I would also consider taking blood cultures and sensitivities. For diagnostic purposes, I would request a breast ultrasound scan in order to identify any underlying abscess which may appear as a hypoechoic lesion. This can be combined with a diagnostic needle aspiration, which would provide symptomatic relief and be useful for diagnostic purposes. The aspirate can be sent away for cytology to ensure there are no malignant changes.

'What features in a mammogram scan would you expect to see for a breast abscess?'

Mammography in breast infection is often quite painful and can be non-specific. However, findings may include increased density of tissue around the infection site, a spiculated mass, calcifications and underlying skin retraction or thickening. When there may be a suspicion of malignancy, it is usually more helpful to perform the mammography after resolution of the acute presentation, ideally in patients aged >40 years old.

'How would you manage this patient, if confirmed to have an acute breast abscess?'

I would ascertain the MRSA status of the patient, and also ensure the patient was not penicillin allergic. I would then initiate antibiotic therapy; this may be intravenous or oral, depending on the severity alongside adequate pain relief. I would review the patient within 48 hours to ensure she is responding to the treatment. If there was a limited response, or the lesion was a well-developed, mature abscess, I would proceed with needle aspiration under ultrasound guidance, if available. This may need to be repeated multiple times over a few days depending on the abscess. I would reserve incision and drainage procedures for those patients in whom aspiration fails, or for very large abscesses – typically more than 5 cm.

Background information

Breast infections are a common abnormality, typically affecting females aged between 15–45 years old and lactating. *Staphylococcus aureus* is the most prevalent skin commensal, and therefore unsurprisingly, is the most commonly isolated pathogen. Early identification and treatment of mastitis is effective in preventing the development of further complications such as a breast abscess. A fistula may be formed when an abscess ruptures with no resolution of the draining sinus. Mastitis may be secondary to lactation, or other disease processes such as duct ectasia.

In lactational mastitis, entry sites from the surface may inoculate the milk present within the breast due to overproduction or milk stasis. Entry sites can be through breaks in the skin, or fissures, with source organisms arising from the skin surface or an infant's oral cavity. In duct ectasia, the lactiferous ducts undergo squamous metaplasia causing blockage, duct dilation and inflammation. This process predisposes to bacterial infections.

Mastitis and breast abscess can be classified as follows:

Type	Description
Mastitis: Lactational	Breast inflammation secondary to breast feeding, with or without infection
Mastitis: Non-lactational	Breast inflammation secondary, with or without infection, unrelated to breast feeding
Subclinical mastitis	Breast milk has signs of mastitis without clinical presentation. This typically includes raised sodium/potassium ratio and interleukin levels
Breast abscess	Localised pus collection contained within granulomatous walls

Clinical vignettes for further practice

A 44-year-old female presents with a new right-sided breast mass. She noticed the mass whilst changing her clothes, but admits to not performing regular self-examinations of her breasts. Upon examination, there is a hard, irregularly shaped mass 2 by 1 cm in the upper outer quadrant of the right breast. There is no accompanying nipple discharge, skin changes or lymphadenopathy.

> You cannot be expected to know every surgical speciality. My experience was mostly in colorectal surgery during my foundation jobs, and I had little experience in subspecialties such as breast and urology, which unfortunately came up during my clinical station. I was able to answer some initial questions but struggled with the more in-depth material. The safest thing to do is to be honest, the interviewer moved onto another area which I was much more confident with, and later in the station came back to the original question.

2.11 BURNS

Clinical case

You are the surgical CT1 on call and are asked to see a 31-year-old male who presents to A/E after spilling hot oil onto his left foot. He immediately washed his foot and his partner wrapped it in cling film. He is otherwise fit and well with no other relevant past medical or surgical history. The emergency team place an antiseptic cream over the foot.

'Describe the clinical photograph.'

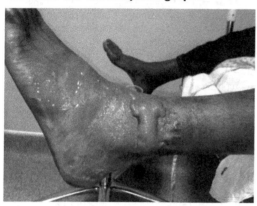

Variable vignettes have been used in the clinical station, though most centre around written vignettes. Presenting clinical photographs, radiographs and other investigations will greatly increase your confidence and breadth of knowledge.

This is a clinical photograph of what appears to be an African-Caribbean patient's left ankle. There is clear blistering over the superior aspect of the lateral malleolus. The area of the blister is large and irregular, with smaller satellite blisters situated above the main site of injury. There are clear, well-demarcated raised edges. There does not appear to be any breaks in the skin or other signs of injury. There is a coating of antiseptic cream over the entire left ankle, which is a grey-white colour.

'How would you classify burns?'

Depth	Description
First degree (Erythema)	Overlying erythema which is painful and dry. Capillary dilation causes erythema, which may or may not be accompanied by blistering.
Second degree (Superficial partial thickness and deep partial-thickness burns)	Burns that involve the epidermis and germinal layer; this is accompanied by blistering and slough formation. In deep partial thickness, the injury involves appendages such as hair follicles and sweat glands. The injury is painful and accompanied by exudation.
Third degree (Full-thickness burns)	Complete destruction of the skin, which appears dry and classically painless with a leathery appearance.
Fourth degree	Subcutaneous tissue, underlying structures such as tendons and bones become visible. Often dry and painless.

'How would you estimate the burn area of the patient's foot in the clinical photograph?'

For this particular patient, I would employ the Lund and Browder classification, which allows accurate burn estimation based on the premise that the patient's palm is of average size. The palm represents approximately 1% of the total body surface area. An alternative system is the Wallace rule of nines by which anatomical segments are given in estimated burn percentages. In accordance with this system, the head and neck represent 9%, and the anterior and posterior thorax region are 18% each. Each lower limb is 18%, while each upper limb is 9%. This system also represents scattered or irregular areas as 1% of the patient's palm.

Burns are a common presentation that requires competent management across all acute specialities involved in its care. The ATLS course provides an excellent approach for patients with acute burns including thermal injuries, hypothermic burns and management protocols.

'What investigations would you undertake for this patient?'

Following resuscitation, I would request a urine analysis with a urine dipstick to screen primarily for renal injury by looking for haematuria and proteinuria. I would request bloods, specifically the FBC, looking for signs of hypovolaemia, and importantly raised WCC and neutropenia indicative of infection. In more serious injuries, I would specifically look at the urea and electrolytes to assess for derangements due to fluid losses. In an inhalational injury, an arterial blood gas and carboxyhaemoglobin level would be helpful.

'How would you treat the patient in the clinical photograph?'

The patient appears to have less than 1% superficial partial thickness burns (or second-degree burns). I would first give the patient analgesic to treat his acute discomfort, as well as that which may follow treatment. I would clean the wound with water and simple soap. I would apply an antibiotic cream, preferably one containing silver – such as topical silver sulfadiazine – to prevent infection. Although there is no obvious sign of skin breach, I would give the patient a tetanus injection if they were not immunised. Finally, I would consider speaking to a surgical subspecialty for further advice.

'Would you refer the patient to a specialist burns centre?'

The current guidelines state that patients who suffer more than 10% total body surface area burns should be referred to specialist burns centres, which would not be appropriate in this patient.

Background information

Burns can be a challenging topic since they are common but their management is often directed towards specialist burns units, although patients are often treated within an A/E setting first. The majority of burns are eventually treated in the community, with a minority suffering from severe burns requiring inpatient care. Young children and elderly patients are the most commonly affected. You must be vigilant in identifying wound infection risks. The most common skin commensal is *Staphylococcus aureus*, and patients who are in an immunocompromised state and receive severe burns can suffer from disastrous consequences.

Specialist investigations include fluorescein staining for corneal injuries and carboxy haemoglobin levels, particularly in cases of inhalational injury. Indications for inpatient care include total surface body area burns exceeding 10%. Oral cavity and thoracic burns limit the patient's ability to consume fluids or breath adequately. An assessment of the patient's competency and compliance must also be carried out. Patients who are unable to control their pain, are unlikely to attend scheduled appointments, present multiple co-morbidities that would limit healing or have severe injuries that demonstrate signs of infection should be considered for admission at burn units.

Fluid resuscitation becomes particularly important in patients with more than 15% burns. The Parkland formula is popularly used to facilitate fluid management, though in most patients the capillary function is restored after 24 hours. The Parkland formula is given as follows:

- 4 mL × kg × % burn for the first 24 hours.
  - The first 50% of this figure should be delivered in the initial 8 hours, usually as a Hartmann's solution.
  - The following 50% should be delivered over the next 16 hours, usually as a Hartmann's solution.
  - Children typically receive 5% dextrose in a Hartmann's solution to prevent the occurrence of hypoglycaemia.
  - In a 70 kg female suffering 10% burns, the fluid requirements in addition to maintenance fluid would be:
    - 4 × 70 × 10 = 2800 mL over 24 hours. This would be delivered as:
- 1400 mL over 8 hours.
- 1400 mL over the remaining 16 hours.

Operative management is reserved for those patients that suffer large areas of full-thickness burns, limb-threatening burns or circumferential burns involving the torso which could limit respiratory effort. An escharotomy procedure over the damaged skin areas can help to alleviate the aforementioned problems. It is important to note that burn complications often arise 12–24 hours after the initial injury, and include limb-threatening ischaemia. Ideally, autografts should be used to close wounds, thus limiting systemic inflammations and sepsis that would otherwise occur.

Clinical vignettes for further practice

A 7-year-old male child is brought into A/E after his mother tripped over, and accidentally spilled hot tea over his right arm. The arm has been covered in emollient cream by the parents and shows blistered skin that has begun to slough away. The burn extends from the elbow, along the dorsum of the forearm to the wrist, and is exquisitely painful.

Practise, practise, practise! I was never one to get into groups or even work in twos when preparing for the surgical interviews. It was only when I joined some friends who were practising and needed a spare interviewer that I realised how robotic and unprepared I sounded. There was a massive difference between my delivery and thought processes, when being interviewed, compared to my friends who were far slicker and well presented.

2.12 CHEST INJURY

Clinical case

A 24-year-old male was involved in a road traffic accident, having lost control of his car and crashed into a wall. The front end of the car suffered significant damage, causing the safety air bags to be deployed. The patient required 20 minutes to be safely extracted from the vehicle. On arrival, the patient is on a spinal board with C-spine immobilisation. The primary survey shows a patent airway with spontaneous breath sounds, however there is an asymmetrical chest expansion on the right-hand side. Upon inspection, bruising from the seat belt can be seen running across the patient's right shoulder obliquely across the chest with exquisite tenderness over the right ribs.

'What thoracic injuries would you be most concerned about?'

Given the history of mechanical force, this patient has been exposed to blunt force trauma. There is bruising over the chest with asymmetrical chest expansion and pain over the ribs. I would therefore be most concerned about the development of a tension pneumothorax. Other injuries I would be concerned about include a haemothorax, flail chest, rib fractures and underlying lung injury such as a contusion.

> Trauma involves prioritising a patient's injuries and then providing focused treatment. When necessary, activate the appropriate teams early, as well as request important investigations without delay.

'How would you recognise a tension pneumothorax?'

I would check to see if the patient's trachea was central and not deviated, and if this was accompanied by distended neck veins. As the patient already has an asymmetrical chest expansion on the right, I would percuss the chest and listen for hyper-resonant percussion notes. On auscultation, I would listen for reduced or absent breath sounds. I would also review the patient's basic observations and ensure that they were not decompensating based on his heart rate, blood pressure and oxygen saturation levels.

'Present this PA chest radiograph.'

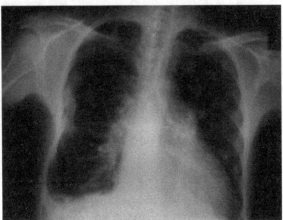

This is a chest radiograph of a rotated patient who has taken an adequate inspiration, and in whom the penetration of the radiograph is adequate. The most obvious abnormality in this radiograph are multiple fractures of the ribs, which are misplaced and impeding into the right lung field. There are no visible lung markings in the right lower lobe of the patient's lung field in close proximity to the damaged ribs, in keeping with a pneumothorax. There is also increased shadowing along the border of the right mediastinum. The trachea is central and not deviated; the mediastinum is normal in size and proportion. The heart appears globular and significantly increased in size. I cannot see any air under the right hemi-diaphragm, subcutaneous air or any other abnormality on this film.

'What is your diagnosis for this patient?'

Given the mechanism of injury and the presence of fractured ribs, which appear to be separate from the bony structure of the lungs, this patient may have suffered from a flail chest injury. Confirmed-the chest radiograph supports the finding, one of the complications of this injury is damage to the underlying viscera. This appears to have occurred resulting in a pneumothorax.

'How would you recognise a flail chest injury clinically?'

A flail chest injury results from the fracture of a rib segment in two places, such that it is no longer part of the bony lung architecture on the ipsilateral side of injury. It is recognisable from paradoxical chest wall movements that are dysynchronous from normal lung movements. I would also look for surrounding chest injuries, such as bruising and lacerations that support blunt force. In order to treat a flail chest, I would ideally give humidified oxygen with titrated oxygen ventilation through a non-rebreather mask. I would provide the patient with adequate analgesic to aid their respiratory effort, and also instigate careful fluid resuscitation.

The patient starts to complain of chest pain. You notice distended neck veins; the chest sounds are clear on both sides, however you have difficulty auscultating the heart sounds. Patient observations are: HR: 60; RR: 24; BP: 80/50 mm Hg; Sats: 88%.

'How would you proceed?'

This patient appears to be suffering from a cardiac tamponade as he is displaying Becks' triad, which includes hypotension, distended neck veins and distant heart sounds. The patient is unstable and I would immediately call for senior surgical help. I would begin resuscitating the patient and place him on high-flow oxygen through a non-rebreather mask. I would re-examine the chest to confirm there is not an alternative cause for the patient's deterioration, and ensure the chest drain contents were swinging. I would proceed to gain intravenous access and send away bloods. At this stage, I would not begin fluid resuscitation until senior support had arrived.

'Your consultant wishes to treat this patient with pericardiocentesis. Do you know any indications for this procedure?'

Pericardiocentesis is one of the options for treating a cardiac tamponade. It is usually reserved for patients who are haemodynamically unstable with a systolic blood pressure below 110 mm Hg and pulsus paradoxus >10 mmg Hg. Positive echo findings that confirm an effusion around the heart, or right ventricular collapse, would also support the use of pericardiocentesis. The presence of aortic dissection is a contraindication against this procedure.

'This patient is hypotensive. What non-haemorrhagic causes of shock do you know?'

Non-haemorrhagic causes of shock include cardiogenic shock, for example secondary to cardiac tamponade, which may include muffled heart sounds, distended neck veins and hypotension. Also, a tension pneumothorax, neurogenic shock, for example in spinal cord damage, which may present with hypotension in the absence tachycardia. And lastly, septic shock which often presents with fever.

Background information

Clinical vignettes involving trauma require strict prioritisation of differentials and management of those that are most life-threatening. Chest trauma is precarious because of the many vital organs that can be effected, thus requiring specific management plans depending on the mechanism of action and likely structures that have been damaged. The ATLS course is highly recommended, as the manual will provide an excellent run-through of trauma situations and all of the clinical knowledge you need for these situations. These clinical scenarios will help you apply this knowledge, and will serve you well in your surgical career whenever on call.

Injury	Presentation	Treatment
Tension pneumothorax	Deviated trachea, asymmetrical chest expansion, hyper-resonant percussion notes, reduced or absent breath sounds	Immediate needle thoracocentesis in the second intercostal space mid-clavicular line of the affected side. Definitive treatment is with chest drain insertion
Haemothorax	Patients may have a deviated trachea in severe injury. Asymmetrical chest expansion, dull percussion notes and reduced breath sounds	Chest drain insertion
Flail chest	Paradoxical chest movements	Humidified oxygen, ventilation support, analgesic and careful fluid resuscitation
Cardiac tamponade	Beck's triad: Hypotension, muffled heart sounds and distended neck veins	Pericardiocentesis
Pulmonary contusion	Guided by history and often accompanies rib fractures and flail chest. Can be diagnosed on CT scan	Ventilatory support

Clinical vignettes for further practice

A 42-year-old male falls from a ladder onto his back. He is conscious on arrival to A/E with C-spine immobilisation. There is a large laceration to the occiput, bruising over the left ribs and a large bruise over the patients left upper quadrant. The patient has a GCS of 15/15 and observations show a tachycardia of 110 bpm and blood pressure 100/77 mm Hg.

Do not be disheartened by the interviewers testing you. I had recently completed the ATLS course and I had an interest in trauma. By the end of the station, I was being quizzed on guidelines in trauma management and quite advanced material. I had worked hard on giving succinct and complete answers during the station, and it's normally a really good sign if you start getting pushed into more advanced material.

2.13 CHEST PAIN

Clinical case

A 19-year-old male presents with acute right-sided chest pain whilst walking to work. He describes the pain as being very sudden, sharp and on the right side of his chest, accompanied by increasing shortness of breath. He denies any other preceding problems including productive cough, fever or trauma to the area. He suffers from no other medical problems and leads a healthy lifestyle with regular exercise. He is tall in height with a lean body habitus. On meeting the patient he appears anxious, mildly short of breath and holding the right side of his chest.

'What are your differentials for this patient?'

This patient has suffered an acute pain in the right side of the chest accompanied by shortness of breath. Given the demographic of the patient and his body habitus, my primary differential would be a spontaneous pneumothorax. I would wish to examine the patient to ensure he was clinically stable. My other differentials would include an acute exacerbation of asthma and an acute muscular pain. Although this is a young and seemingly healthy individual, I would also wish to exclude cardiac pathologies and a pulmonary embolism. Although unlikely they have a high associated morbidity.

Good surgical practice begins with good medicine. Do not ignore relevant medical issues including past medical problems and medications. It can be very easy to focus entirely on surgical management. Use the clinical, psychological and social model of medicine to fully address a patient's ideas, concerns and expectations.

'What investigation would you consider?'

Assuming the patient was clinically stable based on clinical examination, I would wish to confirm my suspicion with an erect chest radiograph. I would be looking for signs of a pneumothorax. This would be evidenced by absent peripheral lung markings, the presence of a visceral pleural outline, atelectasis and a possible loss of volume though many patients are often hyper-expanded due to increased respiratory efforts. Although I would not expect them in this patient, other lung pathologies may be evident on the CXR, which may contribute to the occurrence of a pneumothorax.

'How would you manage a patient with suspected tension pneumothorax?'

I would insert a standard 14-gauge intravenous cannula into the second intercostal space in the mid-clavicular line. I would do this immediately and not depend on any further investigations, including a chest radiography.

I would listen for the hiss of gas release from the cannula and reassess the patient and his vital signs to ensure he is stabilising. I would alert a senior in surgery for urgent patient assessment and definitive management.

'Describe your definitive management if you saw this patient's CXR.'

This patient appears to have a right-sided pneumothorax with right lung collapse. This is evidenced by an absence of lung markings at the periphery of the right lung. Also, there is a clear outline of the right lung separated away from the lung extremity. The trachea appears central and not deviated with no signs of mediastinal shift. For definitive management, I would insert a chest drain on the affected side of the patient's chest. This would be under the supervision of a senior, and following an aseptic technique. I would identify the safe triangle typically at the 5th intercostal space above the rib and in the anterior axillary line. Following blunt dissection, I would aim the chest tube apically for a pneumothorax, or basally for fluid, although the tube's final position is not vital for drainage. I would ensure I had removed the trocar to prevent injury.

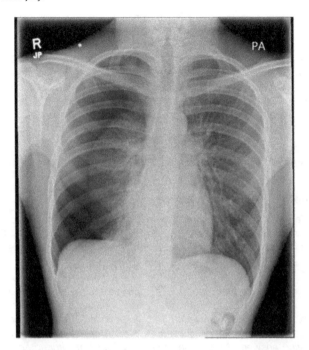

'Following a successful insertion, how would you manage the chest drain?'

After securing the chest, I would examine the patient to check for signs of breathlessness, distress or development of subcutaneous emphysema. I would check the tubing itself to see if any effluent was being produced and then place the drain into a single flow drainage system with an underwater seal. I would check the water to see signs of escaping air from the patients' chest. This would confirm the therapeutic effect of the intervention as well as confirm the patency of the drainage system. Finally, I would ask the patient to cough and check for increased bubbling in the underwater seal. If fluid is draining from the lung, I would see swinging in the chest tube itself.

Background information

A pneumothorax describes the accumulation of gas in the pleural space, most often due to traumas that disrupt the normal pleural architecture. They may be classified as primary or secondary. The former most often occur without any preceding stimulus in patients who are often young (<40), tall, have a lean body habitus, have a family history of pneumothorax, have Marfan's syndrome or smoke cigarettes. Secondary causes arise most often due to important co-morbidities including acute severe asthma due to air trapping, chronic obstructive pulmonary disease – most often due to subpleural bleb rupture, and finally, iatrogenic causes such as a central venous catheter insertion.

Patients may typically present with a range of symptoms and signs including:

- Chest pain ipsilateral to the side of the pneumothorax
- Shortness of breath
- Chest hyper-expansion

- Hyper-resonant tympanic notes on percussion
- Tracheal shift away from the pneumothorax
- Ipsilateral reduced, or absent, breath sounds

In primary spontaneous pneumothoracies, observation and high-flow oxygenation is often sufficient treatment. This is typically for patients with a <2 cm visible dissociation between the lung margin and chest wall. High-flow oxygen, around 10 L/min, has been shown to considerably increase the recovery from pneumothorax. In patients with a >2 cm separation, percutaneous aspiration should be attempted by placing an intravenous cannula at the second intercostal space in the mid-clavicular line with syringe aspiration. Care must be taken to prevent re-entry of air into the pleural space. This should be supplemented with high-flow oxygen to aid recovery. If unsuccessful, a chest drain insertion serves as definitive management.

Secondary spontaneous pneumothorax should similarly receive high-flow oxygenation with definitive management involving the insertion of a chest drain as long as the patient is not unstable.

Clinical vignettes for further practice

A 56-year-old female presents after falling from a ladder. The patient is placed in a C-spine collar, her observations are: HR: 110, RR: 18, BP: 100/80 mm Hg and GCS 13. There is bruising over the right side of the thorax and the patient presents asymmetrical breathing over this side.

> 'During our interview practice, a really helpful technique that we used was to present a scenario to each other and then formulate a question by picking on a topic, disease or investigation that is mentioned in the previous answer. As the person answering the questions, it really makes you firm and precise when giving answers. I mentioned the use of CVP monitoring and instantly regretted it!'

2.14 DEHISCENCE

Clinical case

You are contacted by the ward sister who has become concerned about a 55-year-old female who is recovering from a laparotomy for bowel obstruction. The patient has had a stormy postoperative period complicated by atelectasis, chest infections and ileus. The patient has started to open her bowels but has still not fully recovered from her respiratory discomfort. The patient complains of an abdominal ache and the nurse in charge notices a pink discolouration of the wound dressing. On removal, she is shocked to see open abdominal contents and hurriedly places a stoma bag over the wound. Upon examination, you see the following:

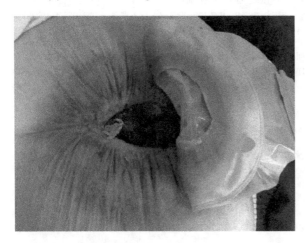

There are various clinical photographs and investigations as practice material. The main purpose behind this is to provide genuine clinical scenarios that challenge you to think based on real-life situations. Candidates have been presented with such material in their stations in the past. This forms an excellent basis for further discussion.

'What has happened to the patient?'

The patient appears to have suffered from a wound dehiscence, sometimes known as a 'burst abdomen'. The original wound incision is present with a central opening, and evisceration of the abdominal contents is visible. There is surrounding erythema around the wound, though no active discharge. The nurse described a pink effusion that is likely to have been serosanguinous fluid known as the 'pink fluid sign', which commonly precedes this pathology.

'What factors can contribute to wound dehiscence?'

I would classify the factors that can contribute to wound dehiscence as preoperative, operative and postoperative. The preoperative factors would include those that impact wound healing and are multifactorial. Operative causes would include a range of factors related to abdominal wound closure. This would include poor surgical technique, such as wound opposition and knot tying, inappropriate suture material choice with poor tensile strength, or poorly placed sutures such as near the wound edge. Excessive tension compounded by inadequate patient relaxation, poor wound healing and complications also contribute to poor closure. Postoperative causes would again include several different factors that raise intra-abdominal pressure. This places pressure upon the margins of the suture line. This can include cough induced by chest infections, atelectasis, asthma and COPD. Pathological causes for abdominal distension such as a paralytic ileus, constipation or haematomas are common following operative management and precipitate this problem. Finally, the integrity of the wound itself can be compromised by infection causing weakening.

'What preoperative factors can affect wound healing?'

There are multiple different factors that can impede optimal wound healing. These include wound infections which disturb the wound architecture and deter fibroblast-led healing. Also, poor oxygenation to the area which can occur from several different causes such as anaemia, respiratory illness, obesity and smoking. Important elements such as vitamin C, A and B6 are all important in collagen production. Finally, certain disease states actively work against adequate wound repair, which include diabetes and corticosteroid use.

'How would you manage this patient?'

I would begin by reassuring the patient who, along with the nursing staff, is likely to have been greatly distressed by their wound complication. I would examine the abdomen and ensure that other compounding factors, such as wound infection or hernias, were not present. I would give the patient analgesic alongside an antiemetic for pain relief and to reduce their anxiety. I would place the patient nil by mouth and apply sterile dressings, or towels soaked in normal saline, and alert my surgical senior. I would begin to make preparations for theatre as definitive management would involve re-closure of the wound, preferably with nylon sutures appropriately placed through all the abdominal wall layers.

Background information

Abdominal wound dehiscence is the partial or complete disassociation of the wound layers, which risks leading to the evisceration of the abdominal organs. Patients are most at risk of this complication when the strength of the wound is weakest, typically between the 8th to 10th postoperative day. Thoracotomy and abdominal repairs are the most common wounds in which dehiscence occurs. The pink fluid sign represents the exudation of serosanguinous fluid, which is often shortly followed by complete wound breakdown. Wound closure is advocated in most patients, however other treatment options include allowing drainage of the infected wounds through a vacuum-assisted drainage and closure at a later, more appropriate date.

Clinical vignettes for further practice

A 24-year-old male is discharged 8 days postoperatively following a successful laparotomy and repair after suffering a penetrating trauma to the abdomen. He returns due to concerns about persistent wound discharge. Upon examination, the laparotomy wound does not appear infected and is mostly intact. There is a small defect in the centre of the wound from which serosanguinous fluid is discharging.

> The interviewers are good at keeping you on track. I remember speaking for quite a long period when answering a question and – panicked – thinking I was wasting time in giving the wrong answer. If you have more useful or relevant things to say, then just keep talking until you are interrupted or moved on.

2.15 DISLOCATED SHOULDER

Clinical case

You are on call and covering for orthopaedics. A 19-year-old male presents to A/E after suffering a fall onto his shoulder while skateboarding. He is fit and healthy and has no relevant medical problems. The A/E department is extremely busy and they escalate the patient to your registrar who accepts and asks you to see him. Upon examination, the patient is in extreme pain but stable and holds his right arm in a slightly abducted and externally rotated position.

'What are your differentials for this patient?'

The patient may have suffered a number of possible injuries, although my primary diagnosis is an anterior shoulder dislocation. The patient has a characteristic history and the arm is held in a typical position suggesting shoulder dislocation, the vast majority of which are anterior. The patient may have suffered a proximal humerus fracture, though this is usually accompanied by bruising and swelling. There may be a clavicle fracture, which is not always obvious on clinical examination. I would also review imaging investigations to check for acromioclavicular joint separation, which commonly accompanies traumatic injuries to the shoulder.

'How would you proceed with this patient?'

I would resuscitate the patient and assess his level of health using the ALS protocol A, B, C. Starting with the airway, I would speak with the patient and ensure there was a patent airway and no escalation was needed. I would briefly examine the chest for any gross pathologies and assess the patient's cardiovascular status. I would gain intravenous access and review adjuncts such as oxygen saturation, ECG and blood pressure monitoring. I would expose the patient and check for any other signs of injury, including limb deformities. I would react to any abnormal clinical findings and initiate therapy, at which point I would reassess the patient. Once the patient is stable, I would then take a focused history based on the patient's presenting complaint and relevant past medical and drug history as well as social circumstances.

'What analgesic would you consider giving to the patient?'

In the acute setting, I would use nitrous oxide combined with oxygen (entonox). In my experience, this provides rapid relief of pain, which the patient is in control of, is easy to use and is not invasive. The side effects are minimal compared to alternatives. Other agents would include intravenous opiate-based analgesic alongside sedation. This is highly effective but usually needs senior supervision, since the side effects include respiratory depression and reduced consciousness after reduction. This can make the post-procedure management more difficult and prolonged. Intra-articular anaesthetic, such as lidocaine 1%, is a safe and effective method when administered laterally at the glenohumeral joint. Although there is a risk of introducing an infection, this method avoids airway management concerns and post-procedure monitoring.

'What investigation would you consider to diagnose the abnormality?'

I am suspecting a shoulder dislocation given the mechanism of injury and characteristic position of the shoulder. I would therefore request an antero-posterior X-ray view of the affected shoulder, ideally with internal and external humeral rotation. For the lateral view, I would request an axillary lateral or shoulder Y-view, which has a high sensitivity for shoulder dislocations.

'How would your investigation help you decide what dislocation had occurred?'

The AP view would typically show the humeral head lying in an anterior and inferior position to the coracoid, often described as the 'light bulb' sign due to the appearance of the head of the humerus. In a posterior dislocation, the humerus head may appear normal and difficult to interpret, thus I would review the axillary view of the shoulder. The scapular Y view would typically show the humeral head to be situated anterior to the 'Y', which is formed by the acromion, coracoid and scapula body in an anterior dislocation. In a posterior dislocation, I would expect the humeral head to be posterior. I could also view the rest of the shoulder radiograph to check for proximal humerus dislocations, clavicle fracture or acromioclavicular joint disruption.

'What injuries are commonly associated with anterior and posterior shoulder dislocations?'

The most common injuries associated with these dislocations are the Bankart and Hill-Sachs lesions. In an anterior shoulder dislocation, the humerus is forced anteriorly, as it does so there is a risk of causing damage to the supporting glenoid labrum and anterior capsule; this is called a Bankart lesion. This usually requires an MRI scan in order to diagnose confidently. In posterior dislocations, the posterior head of the humerus suffers a compression fracture, which is often visible on radiographs and is called a Hill-Sachs lesion.

'Describe the Kocher's technique for shoulder dislocation reduction.'

On the affected limb, the patients' elbow is flexed and adducted against the body. Using a slow and deliberate method the arm is gently externally rotated whilst abducting the forearm. When resistance is felt the forearm is maintained in an externally rotated position and the arm is lifted across the chest, finally, the procedure is ended by internally rotating the forearm so that it is placed on the opposite shoulder.

'What are the complications associated with the Kocher's method of reduction?'

The patient may suffer from humeral shaft fractures, axillary vein rupture and damage to the major muscle groups, such as a pectoralis major rupture.

Background information

Joint dislocation occurs when there is separation between two articulating bony surfaces following traumatic force; joints commonly affected include the shoulder, finger, patella, hip and elbow. Anterior shoulder dislocations are typically held in an externally rotated and abducted position. Conversely, posterior shoulder dislocations are held in adduction and internal rotation. Dislocations are characterised by pain, immobility, tenderness and swelling. Treatment involves analgesic and a safe method of reduction for which there are many techniques including Kocher's, Milch's, Cunningham's, and so forth.

It is essential, after reduction, to obtain an AP and lateral radiograph of the affected shoulder to ensure that successful reduction has taken place and no iatrogenic fractures have occurred. Following recovery from analgesic, a neurological and vascular examination should be carefully performed and documented.

Patients should be placed in a sling for approximately 3 weeks following reduction to aid support and recovery. In young patients below the age of 25, an orthopaedic referral is mandated due to the high risk of recurrence, and there is now a move to initiate primary stabilization through a Bankart's repair.

Clinical vignettes for further practice

A 34-year-old electrician presents to A/E having suffered an electric shock whilst at work. He is fully conscious throughout the event, suffers no chest pain or shortness of breath. However, he was thrown back from the shock and has extreme pain in his left shoulder, which he holds in an adducted and internally rotated position.

Trainee advice

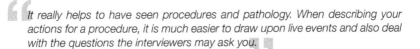

It really helps to have seen procedures and pathology. When describing your actions for a procedure, it is much easier to draw upon live events and also deal with the questions the interviewers may ask you.

2.16 EPIGASTRIC PAIN

Clinical case

You are referred a 60-year-old male who has presented with a 3-hour history of acute severe epigastric pain that radiates to the back. The patient had been drinking when the pain first started and increased rapidly. He has vomited multiple times and constantly changes his posture to relieve the pain, and finds that leaning forward is the most comfortable position. He denies any changes in his bowel habits and, aside from hyperlipidaemia, is fit and healthy. He has been advised to limit his alcohol intake on multiple occasions. His observations are:

HR: 110; Blood pressure: 91/62 mmHg; RR: 22; Sats: 99% on air.

'What are your differentials for this patient?'

My primary diagnosis for this patient includes acute pancreatitis. My other important considerations would include peptic ulcer disease, perforation of an intra-abdominal viscus due to a complication of appendicitis or diverticulitis. I would also consider an abdominal aortic aneurysm, cholecystitis and mesenteric ischaemia.

> Justify your investigations fully – knowing why you are performing each blood test is a common question often very poorly answered by candidates.

'What blood investigations would you consider?'

After resuscitating the patient, I would begin my investigations with an FBC to look for leukocytosis and reduced haematocrit, which is suggestive of pancreatic necrosis. Urea and electrolytes would also be helpful to guide the level of hydration and as a baseline for further investigations. Liver function tests, particularly AST and ALT, would be helpful in suggesting gallstone disease which is a common precipitant of pancreatitis, whilst GGT is suggestive of obstructive causes. Serum lipase is an expensive test that is not always available. It is, however, specific and sensitive for pancreatitis, therefore helpful in eliminating other differentials. If this is not available, serum amylase is a less accurate test, which is affected by other disease states such as alcoholism, hyperlipidaemia and salivary gland inflammation. The arterial blood gas would be an important investigation to review the level of oxygenation and identify any obvious acid-base disturbances, particularly metabolic acidosis associated with a raised lactate. As part of the Imrie prognostic scoring system, I would also review the calcium, serum glucose, albumin and lactate dehydrogenase levels.

'How would you diagnose pancreatitis?'

I would diagnose pancreatitis based on the presence of two out of the three following presentations; the presence of acute abdominal pain focused in the upper abdominal region, appropriately elevated pancreatic enzymes in the serum or urine and abnormal imaging based on ultrasound, CT or MRI.

'What specific clinical signs would you look for on examination?'

I would look for bilateral flank discolouration, known as Grey-Turner's sign, or a similar discolouration over the peri-umbilical area known as Cullen's sign. Both are suggestive of a haemorrhagic pancreatitis and result from bleeding into the retroperitoneal space. I would also look for bruising over the inguinal ligament area, which is known as Fox's sign. Signs of hypocalcaemia may also be present including facial muscle spasm on tapping the facial muscle or Chvostek's sign. Carpopedal spasm on application of a blood pressure cuff may also be present, otherwise called Trosseau's sign.

'What is the Imrie scoring system?'

The Imrie or Ranson scoring system is a prognostic scoring system for pancreatitis that is used in the first 48 hours to predict severe pancreatitis. A score of >2 would indicate an increased chance of severe pancreatitis, with a maximum score of 8. The prognostic factors that are used include:

	Parameter	Value	Point
P	PaO_2 (arterial)	<10 kPa	1
A	Age	>55 years	1
N	WCC	>15	1
C	Calcium (serum)	<2 mmols	1
R	Raised urea	>16.1 mmols/L	1
E	Enzymes (LDH)	>600 units	1
A	Albumin (serum)	<32 g/L	1
S	Glucose (serum)	>10 mmols/L	1

'How would you interpret this abdominal radiograph?'

The most obvious abnormality on this abdominal radiograph appears to be a localised area of bowel in the ascending colon. In a patient with severe pancreatitis, this may represent a sentinel loop. This is an isolated segment of dilated bowel that is usually in close proximity to the pancreas. It usually manifests as gas in the right colon that abruptly stops over the transverse colon. It is thought to represent a localised ileus that is secondary to the nearby inflammation of the pancreas.

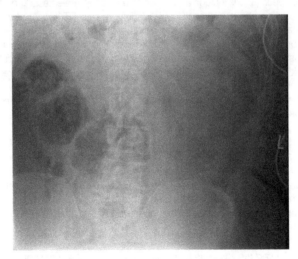

'After resuscitation, what treatment would you initiate?'

I would initiate fluid resuscitation and monitor the urine output closely through catheterisation, ensuring it was above 30 mL/hour. I would prescribe an initial 1 litre fluid bolus followed by 3 mL/kg/hour in the first 24 hours. In patients with heart failure, I would be more careful but still follow an aggressive course of fluid infusion. Alongside this, I would prescribe the patient adequate analgesic and antiemetics, and keep them nil by mouth to rest the bowel and reduce stimulation of the pancreas. If the patient was vomiting profusely, I would also consider inserting a nasogastric tube.

'What adjuncts would you consider in alcohol induced pancreatitis?'

I would be wary of alcoholic patients undergoing withdrawal and therefore would consider prescribing a suitable benzodiazepine. Alongside this, I would consider replacement of thiamine in chronic alcoholic patients.

Background information

Pancreatitis is usually recognised by the classic acute upper-abdominal pain that is constant and radiates to the back. There is often profuse nausea and vomiting, which may be accompanied by fever and sweating. The mainstay of treatment is supportive therapy aimed at preventing worsening of the disease and development of complications.

Up to 20% of patients have an idiopathic cause of pancreatitis though the majority of these patients have some form of biliary disease, such as microlithiasis or biliary sludge. Alcohol is the most common worldwide cause, whilst in the United Kingdom, gallstones are responsible for the majority of presentations. Other important causes include:

- Hypertriglyceridaemia
- Hypercalcaemia
- Infectious (mumps, EBV, HIV)
- Pharmacological (azathioprine, furosemide, oestrogens)
- Iatrogenic most commonly post ERCP
- Trauma
- Pancreatic neoplasm
- Autoimmune disease of the collagen or vascular systems

Accompanying investigations include a CXR, which may show atelectasis and left-sided pleural effusions, and also an ultrasound scan, which is inferior to a CT scan, but which may show signs of pancreatic inflammation, such as peri-pancreatic fat stranding, fluid and calcification. CT scan with contrast is the most sensitive study demonstrating pancreatic dysmorphology, fat necrosis and pseudocysts. Patients on prolonged IV fluid managements should have dietary advice input with feeding considerations, including nasojejunostomy and parenteral nutrition. Patients with gallstone pancreatitis should ideally undergo a cholecystectomy operation in the same admission following stabilisation to reduce recurrence. Necrotic pancreatic tissue may require a necrosectomy and even debridement in case of multi-organ failure and CT evidence of necrosis.

Clinical vignettes for further practice

A 65-year-old female with known gallstones presents with severe upper-abdominal pain radiating to her back. She complains of nausea, vomiting and loss of appetite. She suffers from diabetes, hypertension and hyperlipidaemia but denies heavy drinking or smoking. Upon examination, her abdomen is exquisitely tender around the epigastrum, and you notice a blue discolouration of the umbilical area.

> *I underestimated the investigations in surgical disease and I did not focus much revision as to why I would choose particular investigations. This turned out to be a major hole in my revision. My interviewer asked me why I picked CT scanning over US for pancreatitis and I couldn't give a reasonable answer.*

2.17 EPISTAXIS

Clinical case

You are asked to see a 49-year-old male who has had an uncontrollable nosebleed in A/E. He reports bleeding initially from the right nostril whilst in a business meeting, and then attending the hospital when he wasn't able to control it after 1 hour. He has a blood-soaked towel with him and occasionally has to spit blood into it. He suffers from hypertension and asthma, but is otherwise in good health. His observations are:

Heart rate: 90 bpm; Blood pressure: 160/95 mmHg; RR: 16; Sats: 98%.

'What differentials would you consider for patient?'

The primary diagnosis appears to be an uncontrolled epistaxis. However, I would want to examine the patient and ensure this wasn't masking another pathology, such as haemoptysis or haematemesis. In both situations, a closer examination of the patient is likely to show the nose as the origin of the bleeding.

> Epistaxis is a common presentation during a surgical on-call. This can be challenging, as there is limited exposure amongst trainees, even after medical school.

'What can cause epistaxis to occur?'

The majority of epistaxis episodes occur from a collection of blood vessels in Little's area which collate together forming Kiesselbach's plexus. The majority of bleeding is therefore anterior. Posterior bleeding may occur from the posterior nasal cavity, or nasopharynx, and is often more severe. Vessels may become exposed if there is a breach in the mucosal layer, dysfunction of vasoconstriction or disruption of clotting mechanisms. Hypertension is often associated with epistaxis as well as trauma and anticoagulation abuse.

'What are the important risk factors for epistaxis?'

Epistaxis is often precipitated by reduced humidity and colder climates, which cause loss of moisture in the nasal mucosal layer leading to cracks and breaches. Oxygenation via the nasal cannulae similarly can cause drying of the nasal mucosa. Preceding nasal trauma, including over-zealous nose blowing, can also cause damage and subsequent bleeding. Finally, medical conditions such as coagulopathy, hereditary haemorrhagic telangiectasia and angiofibromas are also causative factors.

'After resuscitation, what features would you look for on examination?'

I would examine for signs of anterior nasal bleeding by looking for haemorrhage at the nares. For posterior nasal bleeding, I would also check the throat. Anterior nose bleeding can present in the back of throat if the patient is supine. I would check the position of the nasal septum, as a deviation can complicate packing insertion. Finally, I would check for sensation impairment in the distribution of the trigeminal nerve, which would suggest malignancy.

'How would you treat this patient?'

I would ensure that all reversible causes such as coagulopathy had been investigated and reversed. I would use a nasal decongestant spray, such as oxymetazoline, to begin vasoconstriction of the blood vessels. After application, I would apply pressure over the compressible area of the cartilage. If this failed, I would use a topical anaesthetic, such as 4% lidocaine, applied to nasal pledgets, or cotton balls alongside the decongestant spray. I would use bayonet forceps to gently insert the nasal packs or cotton balls into the nose and maintain them for 15 minutes.

'What other measures would you try if this failed?'

In more resistant cases, silver nitrate cautery can be used if the bleeding site is easy to visualise. I would apply it to the area of epistaxis, and then place an area of petroleum jelly over the area to protect and maintain moisture. I would warn the patient that the cautery is likely to feel uncomfortable. I would avoid placing the cautery in the same location at either side of the septum, as this can cause septal ischaemia and possible perforation. I would use nasal packing in most cases of active anterior nasal bleeds, and give cover antibiotics against staphylococcus aureus to limit the introduction of infections.

Background information

As described, epistaxis is a common presentation and typically affects those in the young and elderly age bracket. Identification of important risk factors such as coagulopathy, trauma and sites of bleeding – such as nasal polyps – are important to expedite treatment. Although rare from epistaxis alone, you should ensure that you resuscitate the patient every time and check for signs of cardiovascular compromise such as tachycardia, pallor, hypotension, dizziness and collapse. Other investigations are similarly aimed towards identifying aberrant causes of nasal bleeding. These include FBC (anaemia), LFTs (suspected severe hepatic disease), coagulation (severe epistaxis which may be due to coagulopathy) and nasal endoscopy (helpful when diagnosing aberrant bleeding sources or malignancy).

If the aforementioned treatment options fail with silver nitrate cautery, then ENT referral is usually advised since they are more experienced in delivering further treatment such as electrocautery. Nasal packing is an important treatment option that is effective in controlling most bleeding instances. New expanding nasal sponges are now available, which are inserted into a patient's nasal passages and – with the injection of normal saline – expanded to control bleeding. In severe uncontrolled bleeding, lidocaine with adrenaline can be injected into the bleeding site – strictly under experienced hands since it can cause catastrophic complications, including blindness. Posterior bleeding that is not controlled may be treated endoscopically. The most severe instances of uncontrolled bleeding may require open surgical ligation.

Clinical vignettes for further practice

A 9-year-old female with recurrent nose bleeds attends A/E after an episode of uncontrolled epistaxis whilst at school. The mother states she was accidentally hit in the face by another child and used paper towels to control bleeding, but was unable to do so. Upon examination, the child looks well and clinically stable, a bleeding vessel can be seen in the anterior septal mucosa.

> *I was completely caught out at my interview. As silly as it sounds, I focused virtually all of my revision in general surgery and I was very confident with emergencies and acute abdomens. My case scenario was a general surgery topic, which I found easy, but the interview was a nightmare. The second examiner asked me as many questions about orthopaedics and ENT that I couldn't answer, while the first interviewer focused on general surgery. I was completely thrown off by the specialty questions and lost my confidence. Even on questions I was more confident with, I could not answer as well as I normally would have.*

2.18 FOREIGN BODY

Clinical case

You are asked to review a 49-year-old female patient who initially presented to the A/E department with signs of psychiatric instability. Following discharge from the acute mental health team, the patient continues to complain of right iliac fossa pain. The patient denies any difficulty swallowing, shortness of breath or drooling. Upon examination, there are multiple scars and incision sites on the abdomen. There is a horizontal abdominal wound which appears to have been operated on before, and is partially open. The wound is tender on palpation. Previous discharge summaries indicate the patient has a history of self-harm with foreign bodies.

'How would you proceed with this patient?'

I would begin by resuscitating the patient and assess her level of health using the ALS protocol A, B, C, alongside nursing assistance. I would ensure the patient had a patent airway and did not need escalation. I would examine the chest for gross pathologies. For circulation, I would ensure there was intravenous access along with vital sign adjuncts, including oxygen saturation, ECG and blood pressure monitoring. I would consider sending routine blood investigations including FBC, U&E, LFTs and CRP. I would examine the patient's cardiovascular system and assess their haemodynamic status based on capillary refill, presence of pallor, pulse rate, rhythm and nature and praecordium examination findings. I would ensure the patient was properly exposed and, with a chaperone present, I would examine the patient for any other signs of injury. I would react to any abnormal clinical findings and initiate therapy, at which point I would reassess the patient.

'What are you concerned about in this patient?'

Although the patient has been discharged from the acute mental health team, there is a history of self-harm and an injury to the abdomen. I would be concerned about occult injuries the patient may have caused herself, and in particular if she has ingested or inserted foreign objects. This can often range from puncture wounds and lacerations to inserting unusual objects such as metallic items, pencils, batteries and so forth. I would ask specifically about non-specific abdominal pain, bowel habits and PR bleeding.

'Present this clinical photograph.'

This is a clinical photograph of a caucasian patient's abdomen. There is a horizontal wound in close proximity to the umbilicus and it is partially open medially. There appear to be signs of surgical closure and the wound may have dehisced, or forcibly exposed. There is no active discharge from the wound but swab material is visible and soaked at the medial aspect of the wound site. There does not appear to be any surrounding erythema, although there are multiple vertical incisions that do not represent surgical scars.

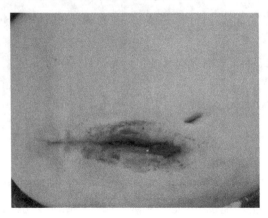

'What investigations would you consider in this patient?'

I would request a urine dipstick to look for haematuria and proteinuria, as a screen for any renal disease. I would check the FBC, urea and electrolytes to look for signs of anaemia, raised WCC, neutrophils and deranged renal function. This may represent occult or active bleeding, as well as reactions to foreign material in the patient. I would also consider faecal occult blood testing as an adjunct to PR examination for foreign bodies potentially in the colorectal system. I would next request chest and abdominal radiographs to look for any obvious signs of foreign bodies. Although the patient denies any symptoms of ingestion, if missed this can be fatal and difficult to manage. I would also wish to further explore the abdomen, as there is an obvious superficial injury which may have caused underlying visceral damage.

'Other than the foreign body, what else would you look for on the chest radiograph?'

I would be most concerned about signs of perforation to the lung. I would look for signs of a pneumothorax, such as a visible pleural outline separate from the peripheral chest wall, absent lung markings and possible tracheal deviation. I would also look for mediastinal damage, which may be represented by enlarged mediastinal borders. I would examine the soft tissues to look for signs of a subcutaneous emphysema, and finally the lung fields for signs of a pleural effusion.

'Present this abdominal radiograph.'

This is an abdominal radiograph that shows normal and unremarkable bowel gas distribution with no signs of obstruction, dilatation or obvious injury. There is no sign of perforation and the most obvious abnormality appears to be several highly attenuated objects in the right iliac fossa, in keeping with the clinical injury on abdominal examination. The objects appear to range from variously shaped screws and sharp objects which are most likely to be in the subcutaneous tissue given their close distribution. The bony architecture appears normal.

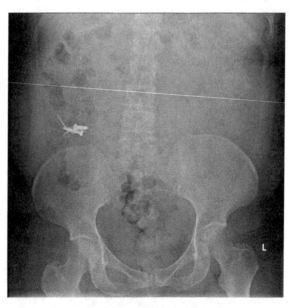

Background information

Foreign body insertion or ingestion is a surprisingly common surgical presentation and ranges from accidental ingestion in children to deliberate self-harm. The majority of ingested foreign material passes through the gastrointestinal system with minimal mucosal injury, however this must be carefully weighed against the risk of bowel obstruction, perforation, haemorrhage and the development of sepsis. Endoscopy now plays an important role in the removal of foreign objects, although it is technically challenging.

Patients showing signs of drooling should have nasogastric or orogastric tube insertion in order to reduce the risk of aspiration. Unstable patients should be resuscitated, and – if there are signs of obstruction or perforation – prepared for operative management. Magnets represent a special subclass of foreign body since they can attract adjacent lying bowel and cause multiple complications including obstruction, fistula formation and pressure necrosis.

Clinical vignettes for further practice

You are asked to review a 5-year-old child who was witnessed ingesting several coins. The mother is extremely anxious and tried to force the child to vomit the foreign bodies at the time of the incident. The child appears well with no signs of distress, but is unusually quiet and drooling constantly.

> *Do not forget your basics! I tried too hard in my interview and spoke about CT guidelines in trauma. The interviewer stopped me during my answer and asked me if I would do a urine dipstick first!*

2.19 GI BLEED

Clinical case

Whilst in the operating theatre, your FY1 colleague accepts a patient for review. He/she presents a 58-year-old female who complains of a 1-month history of epigastric pain and passing darkened stools. The pain has become constant, more severe and the patient points to the epigastrum, describing it as a gnawing pain. The patient suffers from GORD and hypothyroidism. She takes over-the-counter antacids, but states her pain has recently become more painful. She is a chronic smoker and drinks alcohol socially.

'What could this patient be suffering from?'

My primary diagnosis would be peptic ulcer disease given the location of the pain in the epigastrum, and its description in the history alongside the presence of possible malaenia. I would also wish to consider acute pancreatitis, though this would typically present more acutely and does not cause discolouration of the stools. The patient may also have an exacerbation of her gastro-oesophageal reflux disease, although the pain is typically described as a retrosternal burning pain.

> Interviewers will always challenge your answers if not given in a logical manner. Place more exotic diseases, such as Zollinger–Ellison, towards the end of your answer since they are far less common. Even if you are happy to speak at length about the condition, common things are common, therefore present them as such.

'What are the risk factors for peptic ulcer disease?'

Peptic ulcer disease is precipitated by an *H. pylori* infection, the treatment of which is essential in preventing recurrence of disease. Disease may be linked to the use of NSAID medications and corticosteroids are other risk factors. Smoking is another important risk factor although its pathophysiology is unclear.

'What other features in the history would you ask about?'

I would also ask the patient more thoroughly about their NSAID, appetite and smoking habits since these are important risk factors for peptic ulcer disease. Symptoms of anaemia such as shortness of breath, malaise and comments of pallor would be important to identify possible bleeding. The darkened stools would also merit more attention as to their frequency, colour and odour – from which malaenia can be characterised. I would ask about the presence of nausea, vomiting and early satiety, since these can be suggestive of pyloric stenosis. Diarrhoea can present with peptic ulcer bleeding but may also be suggestive of an insidious disease such as Zollinger–Ellison syndrome.

'What are the potential sources of an upper GI bleed?'

There are multiple anatomical locations from which a patient may suffer an upper GI bleed, this can present with haematemesis or as malaenia. Oesophageal varices can present as torrential bleeding, and is usually associated with portal hypertension and liver disease. A Mallory–Weiss tear can also present as an acute episode of upper GI bleeding, and typically involves a period of retching or vomiting violently. Peptic ulcer disease manifests secondary to gastric or duodenal ulcers, the latter being more common and usually associated with *H. pylori*, whilst chronic NSAID use causes gastric ulceration.

'Other than haemorrhage, what other complications are you worried about in peptic ulcer disease?'

Other complications of peptic ulcer disease would include penetration of the ulcer into the surrounding adjacent structures such as the pancreas. This may occur without full perforation and therefore medical treatment is mandated, although surgery may be needed if penetration is severe. Following this perforation, the ulcer erodes through the gastric or duodenal wall with access into the peritoneal cavity. Duodenal and gastric antrum ulcers are most often associated with perforations, and require emergency surgery. Gastric outlet obstruction is usually the result of chronic pyloric stenosis, as ulcers heal with scar formation. Patients may present with nausea, vomiting and on examination a succussion splash may be present.

'The patients' full blood count shows a profound anaemia, what treatment options are available?'

This patient may be suffering from an actively bleeding peptic ulcer. I would therefore ensure that precipitants, such as NSAIDs and aspirin, had been stopped and a suitable PPI had been given. Endoscopic adrenaline injection is an effective treatment as well as allowing confirmation of a bleeding point. Cautery or clip application is often used alongside this to control a bleeding vessel. If endoscopy fails to gain control, the patient should be prepared for operative intervention.

Background information

Peptic ulceration is closely related to dyspeptic symptoms and *H. pylori* and NSAID use represent important causative factors. Factors associated with high bleeding risk and mortality include:

- Age >60
- Anaemia with Hb <8.0
- Shock on admission
- Previous bleeding requiring blood transfusion
- Nasogastric effluent showing ongoing haemorrhage
- Ulcer base showing visible bleeding vessel
- Bright red blood present at ulcer base
- Adherent clot at ulcer base

Red flag signs for prompt endoscopy investigation include patients suffering from significant weight loss, early satiety, anaemia, haemorrhage or dysphagia.

In uncomplicated disease, duodenal ulcers heal in 4 weeks whilst gastric ulcers require a longer period of recuperation, typically healing within 8 weeks. Following eradication of *H. pylori*, patients have a 20% risk of ulcer recurrence. Ulcers associated with NSAID use have a much lower rate of recurrence on the premise that NSAIDs are stopped, or suitable alternatives are sought.

Clinical vignettes for further practice

A 64-year-old male presents to A/E in an intoxicated state. He is known to suffer from osteoarthritis and commonly attends A/E for lower-back pain. Despite advice, he is not compliant with PPI medication and regularly requests repeats for NSAID medication. You receive a fast bleep to attend the resuscitation suite as the patient becomes pale, clammy and sweaty before vomiting a large volume of fresh blood. Upon examination, he is clinically shocked with a rigid, peritonitic abdomen.

Trainee advice

Revising for the MRCS is often helpful in recalling details and facts about surgical disease. Good surgery starts with good medicine and it can be easy to get fixated on just the interventions. Some basic knowledge in the medical physiology and treatment of surgical diseases can be really helpful.

2.20 HAEMATURIA

Clinical case

A 61-year-old male presents with a 2-week history of painless frank haematuria. He has been treated recently for a presumed urinary tract infection, and on first seeing the blood assumed it was the infection clearing itself. He has noticed becoming shorter of breath during the last few months. He denies dysuria and urgency but admits to frequency, waking up several times a night to urinate. He is otherwise well and has no other relevant medical history. He is a social alcohol drinker and is a chronic smoker of 20 cigarettes for 35 years.

Upon examination, the urine is positive for haematuria only and does not contain clots. A PR examination reveals a moderately enlarged, smooth prostate. His observations are:

BP: 130/85 mmHg; Heart rate: 80; RR: 14; Sats: 99% on air.

'What is your primary diagnosis and differentials?'

My primary differential in this patient would be a bladder carcinoma, based on the painless nature of the haematuria alongside important urinary symptoms such as nocturia. The patient is at risk based on his age and smoking history. I would also consider important differentials such as benign prostatic hypertrophy, renal malignancy, prostate cancer and improving urinary infection.

What specific features in the history would you elicit?

As part of my focused history for bladder carcinoma, I would characterise the nature of the haematuria. This would include the presence of clots, in which segment of the urinary flow the haematuria is noticed, for example beginning, middle, end or throughout. I would enquire about the patient's urinary habits including abnormal frequency, urgency, nocturia, dysuria and strength of stream. I would also try to identify important risk factors that may have predisposed the patient to bladder carcinoma including:

- Cigarette smoking
- Exposure to chemical carcinogens
- Pelvic radiation
- Chemotherapy
- Family history

'What investigations would you consider for this patient?'

Once the patient is stabilised, I would confirm the urine analysis to look for proteinuria, leukocytes, nitrites, glucose and ketones. Although the patient is presenting with frank haematuria, this may be mistaken for discolouration. I would therefore confirm the findings with urine analysis. I would then send the sample away for urine microscopy, cytology and sensitivities. I would then consider blood investigations, including an FBC, to look for anaemia and infection. Also, urea and electrolytes analyses to examine for deranged renal function, and liver function tests which specifically include raised ALP – common in bony metastases and hence preclude a bone scan. I would consider an ECG to determine physiological stresses on the heart, which can occur in severe anaemia. A CXR would be important for preoperative considerations and, although unlikely in this patient, render metastases visible. Finally, a cystoscopy investigation would be ideal to visualise a tumour.

'What first line treatment would you consider in a high-risk but non-invasive tumour?'

I would suggest a transurethral resection to treat the carcinoma as well as providing symptomatic relief for episodes of frequency, urgency and haematuria, among others. Once the patient is optimised following this, I would then consider postoperative intravesical chemotherapy such as mitomycin. In a patient with severely obstructive symptoms, a concurrent transurethral resection of the prostate can be performed as this also reduces recurrence.

Background information

Egypt, Western Europe and North America are found to have the highest rates of bladder carcinoma, whilst this is less common in Asian countries. Frank or microscopic haematuria is the most common primary presentation in affected patients, and is often mismanaged as a urinary tract infection.

Central to the diagnosis is the combination of cystoscopy and urine cytology. Low grade tumours are easy to visualise but often have negative cytology. In contrast to this, higher-grade tumours can be more difficult to see due to their flattened appearance, however, they more often appear positive in urinary cytology. Treatment centres around the degree of invasion. In a pathology that spares the detrusor muscle, transurethral resection is the management of choice; although effective, there is a high rate of recurrence. Intravesical chemotherapy is employed in order to reduce the distribution of malignant cells or 'seeding'. In higher grade, more aggressive tumours that have not crossed the detrusor muscle, immunotherapy – using the tuberculosis vaccine BCG – is used with close follow-up. In patients who have muscle-invasive tumours, neoadjuvant chemotherapy, cystoprostatectomy and the surrounding pelvic lymph nodes undergo lymphadenectomy.

Other investigations to consider include:

Investigation	Justification
Ultrasound scan	This can help visualise upper urinary tract and bladder lesions
Intravenous pyelogram	Filling defects caused by bladder malignancy are identified, more detailed than US
CT urogram	More detailed than US, and can aid staging via lymph node detection
MRI	An alternative to CT in patients suspected of having detrusor invasive carcinoma at cystoscopy.

Clinical vignettes for further practice

A 66-year-old female presents with gross haematuria. She has noticed in the last few months significant weight loss, malaise, shortness of breath and recently pains in her joints. She initially suspected a urine infection, and has been treated for this several times during the year. She suffers from hypertension and is a heavy smoker. She became concerned on noticing clots in her urine.

> *I was lucky enough to have a clinical scenario that worked in my favour. I had an interest in urology and naturally read around this subject area more than others. Following a similar format to what you would do when seeing a patient whilst on-call is the best way to predict and practise the type of questions that are asked. This helped me answer the non-urology questions. As you progress further in the station, they can become more challenging but this is generally a good sign.*

2.21 HEAD INJURY

Clinical case

A 43-year-old male attends A/E following an assault at his local pub. He is unable to recall the full events of the evening, but states he became involved in an altercation and was struck on the head from behind. The A/E team clear the patient's C-spine and asks for your assistance.

The patient opens his eyes in response to his name; he is alert but answers in a confused manner. He displays normal motor function. His observations are within normal limits.

'What is this patient's Glasgow coma scale score?'

Based on the patient's ability to open his eyes in response to pain, confused speech and normal motor function his GCS score at present is 13/15, which suggests mild brain injury. I would follow a focused history with a full cranial nerve examination, upper limb and lower examination with a view to request a CT scan of the head.

> A clinical vignette can allow multiple different discussions to take place. The interviewers usually have a specified number of questions, which they must ask in order to compare your responses to other candidates. These are often easy to deduce from the vignette and are usually based on common presentations, investigations and managements as a surgical trainee.

GCS	Eyes	Voice	Movement
1	No response	No response	No response
2	Opens eyes to pain	Incomprehensible sounds	Abnormal extensor response to pain
3	Opens eyes to voice commands	Inappropriate words	Abnormal flexor response to pain
4	Opens eyes spontaneously	Confused vocalisation	Withdraws away from painful stimulus
5		Orientated coherent speech	Localisation towards painful stimulus
6			Spontaneous movement compliant

'During your clinical assessment, what signs are you looking for in a patient with head injury and what pathology do they indicate?'

There are a number of clinical signs I would examine for in this particular patient. Upon inspection, I would look around the eyes for the 'Racoon eye sign'. This is suggestive of periorbital ecchymosis which would result from blood exudation secondary to a basilar skull fracture, particularly in unilateral presentations. I would also inspect the patient's mastoid process for similar signs of ecchymosis. This again can result from blood pooling as a result of basilar skull fractures, and is most often associated with trauma to the petrous part of the temporal bone, which I would palpate for signs of injury. I would move on to examine the ears for signs of bloody otorrhoea, which are also often associated with trauma to the petrous part of the temporal bone. Finally, I would gently palpate around the head for a 'step off', or discrepancy, in the bone architecture which would suggest a fracture.

'How would you confirm the presence of CSF fluid?'

In patients with positive otorrhoea or rhinorrhoea, I would collect a sample and document the time, location and description of the exuded fluid. CSF tends to present as clear fluid or with a mild bloodstained appearance. I would request a beta-2 transferrin immunoassay to test for CSF protein. This has a near 100% sensitivity and specificity for CSF and would direct my suspicions of a CSF leak.

'What neurological signs on the face would you expect in a basilar skull fracture?'

As part of my neurological examination, I would try to elicit signs of sensation deficits or parasthesia suggestive of injury to cranial nerve V. I would also examine for facial paralysis, nystagmus and sensorineural hearing loss, which would suggest damage to cranial nerve VII. These are often closely associated with basilar skull fractures.

'Why is it important to recognise signs of a basilar skull fracture?'

This type of fracture is in close proximity to several cranial nerve structures including the oculomotor, facial and vestibulocochlear nerves. There is also the risk of structures passing through the foramen magnum such as the vertebral arteries, medulla and spinal arteries which, if damaged, would result in catastrophic complications. Basilar skull fractures are the most difficult to identify on a CT scan of the brain, and therefore it is important to identify clinical signs in all patients with traumatic head injury.

'What are the indications for a CT scan of the brain in trauma?'

I would consider a CT scan investigation in patients who present with initial GCS scores below 13, or in patients who have a fluctuant GCS score over a 2-hour period of observation. Other indications include a traumatic mechanism of injury causing a skull fracture, post-event seizure, repeated episodes of vomiting, amnesia exceeding 30 minutes before the traumatic episode or focal neurological deficits.

'A CT scan is performed showing a right frontal haemorrhagic contusion. How does this fit with a patient who was struck at the occiput?'

The CT scan image shows an area of high attenuation at the right frontal lobe, suggesting a recent haemorrhage with an area of oedema around it. There is also signs of attenuation at the left posterior occipital region, which fits with the patient's history of being struck from behind. The impact from behind is likely to have caused the brain to move in the opposite direction and strike the front of the cranium. This has caused haemorrhage, bruising and oedema. The occipital attenuation represents the coup, whilst the area of haemorrhage in the opposite area of the brain represents the contre-coup of the brain injury.

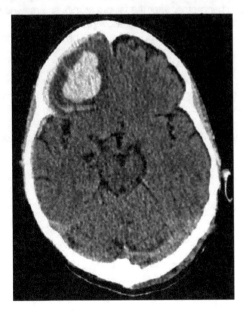

'The neurosurgical unit advises non-operative treatment of this patient. What conservative management would you start?'

The majority of patients with head injury require neurological observation and monitoring. I would admit this patient to be observed for any ongoing complications such as CSF leaks, seizures or fluctuating GCS scores. I would advise the nursing staff to perform regular neurological observations including level of consciousness, pupillary reaction, vital signs, sensory function and motor function.

Background information

Head injury most commonly arises from accidental falls or involvement in high impact injuries such as road traffic accidents and assault. Operative management is more importantly associated with the level and degree of intracranial pathology rather than the fractures incurred.

Common signs of trauma, other than those already mentioned, include soft-tissue swelling in the areas of injuries, bruising, cuts and lacerations. Pooling of blood resulting in haematomas is more suggestive of skull fractures; however, the absence of these signs does not eliminate the possibility of a skull fracture. CT scanning is the mainstay of investigation, alongside the indications already mentioned, and patients who have suffered amnesia exceeding 30 minutes before the trauma are eligible for a CT scan, if any of the following are also present:

* Age >65
* Coagulopathies
* Fall from a height exceeding 3 feet or 5 stairs
* Mechanism of injury involves high force, e.g. road traffic accidents

Post-traumatic seizures are common following a head injury, and although not recommended in isolated skull fractures, prophylactic anticonvulsant therapy such as phenytoin is currently recommended only in open depressed skull fractures, or patients with underlying brain injury.

Clinical vignettes for further practice

A 9-year-old female presents to A/E after having a witnessed fall from a climbing frame at school, approximately 2 metres from the ground. She is fully conscious and stood up immediately, running to her mother after the fall but admits she may have been unconscious for a few seconds. Although teary the patient allows you to examine her head, you palpate a diffuse swelling over the right temporal bone and see a bruise situated over the right mastoid process.

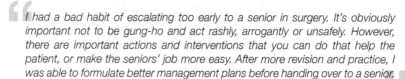

> *I had a bad habit of escalating too early to a senior in surgery. It's obviously important not to be gung-ho and act rashly, arrogantly or unsafely. However, there are important actions and interventions that you can do that help the patient, or make the seniors' job more easy. After more revision and practice, I was able to formulate better management plans before handing over to a senior.*

2.22 HERNIA

Clinical case

You are asked by the paediatric team to review an 8-month-old African-Caribbean male who has been brought into the hospital because of a lump found by his parents. He had a normal uncomplicated birth and has been developing normally. He has had a mild cough and in the morning, whilst bathing, the mother noticed a soft lump protruding at the umbilicus. On examination there is a soft, oval-shaped mass at the umbilicus which does not seem painful.

'What are your differentials for this patient?'

Given the age and examination findings of this child, my primary diagnosis would be an umbilical hernia. I would confirm this by performing a full clinical examination of the abdomen. Other possibilities are limited, although an epigastric hernia would present similarly at the upper abdomen, however defects can be multiple. An omphalocele is seen at birth, and involves the protrusion of the abdominal contents through an umbilical defect with a thin layer of amnion externally, and peritoneum internally.

> Children are not small grown-ups. Their requirements are entirely different to adults, with a subset of presentations. As a core surgical trainee, you will be asked to assess children for a number of pathologies, including appendicitis and hernias.

'What is a hernia?'

This is the protrusion of a viscus through a defect in the containing wall such that the viscus situates in a new and abnormal position covered by its original layers.

'What features would you examine this patient for?'

I would inspect the patient's abdomen to look for a bulge at the umbilicus with intact overlying skin. I would ask them to cough to observe an increase in the size of the bulge. In this patient, I would examine to see the same changes on movement, straining or crying. On palpation, I would examine the skin layer to look for signs of elastication, whether the mass is soft, and importantly, whether it is reducible. Whilst reducing, I would also attempt to determine the size of the defect, which is often a well-defined rim representing the defect.

'What features in the history and examination would worry you?'

I would be concerned by the presentation of obstructive symptoms and signs. These would be nausea, vomiting, abdominal pain and constipation. On examination, if the child appeared unwell, dehydrated and listless, I would be extremely concerned with a low threshold for immediate escalation. Upon examination, an irreducible hernia which was hard, erythematous and exquisitely painful would be suggestive of a strangulated hernia, which is a surgical emergency.

'What would be the management of a tender incarcerated hernia?'

With senior surgical supervision, a tender umbilical mass, with or without signs of strangulation, requires reduction. This can be attempted manually if there are no signs of peritonitis and the patient is clinically stable. Using gentle but firm palpation, air or fluid is coaxed out of the incarcerated bowel, alongside consistent pressure against the mass in an attempt to successfully reduce it. If successful, the patient will need to be admitted and observed for signs of decompensation due to peritonitis. Preparation for defect repair should be made as soon as possible. If this fails, the patient will require operative management and assessment of bowel viability.

'What would be the management of a small, asymptomatic hernia?'

Small hernias that are not causing any discomfort should be kept under observation through patient education, and follow-up is typically until the age of 4–5. The majority of such small hernias spontaneously regress and close. If this does not occur, an elective hernia repair can be organised.

Background information

Paediatric umbilical hernias typically close by the age of 4–5 without intervention; however, although complications are rare they must be recognised and acted on immediately. The umbilicus transmits the contents of the umbilical cord via a defect in the linea alba. The umbilical ring usually closes by contraction, the umbilical vein fibroses to become the round ligament of the liver, and attaches to the umbilicus. This provides anchorage to the umbilicus and protects against the formation of a hernia, however, a minority of patients are susceptible to hernia formation if this process does not occur correctly. Important risk factors for umbilical hernia formation include:

- Low birth weight
- African ancestry
- Trisomy 13, 18 and 21
- Congenital hypothyroidism
- Hurler's syndrome
- Beckwith-Wiedemann syndrome

A large or symptomatic hernia with fascial defects exceeding 1.5–2 cm is unlikely to close naturally. In these patients, earlier intervention at age 2–3 is advocated.

Clinical vignettes for further practice

You are asked to urgently review a 3-year-old male who has presented to A/E with nausea, vomiting and extreme abdominal pain. The child looks dehydrated and unwell, there is a tender mass at the umbilicus, which the child refuses to allow you to examine. His parents state he has not opened his bowels since the morning and has been seen straining constantly during the day.

> *Address both of the interviewers during each question. It might seem really obvious but they tend to ask their own questions and it can be easy in the middle or towards the end of the station to just concentrate on the interviewer posing the particular question.*

2.23 ISCHAEMIC BOWEL

Clinical case

A 66-year-old female presents to A/E after suffering from acute diffuse abdominal pain. The pain started soon after her evening meal and has worsened considerably in the last 6 hours. She had felt reasonably well before this but had noticed abdominal pains around meal times, and thus had avoided eating large meals – resulting in weight loss. She suffers from hypertension, hyperlipidaemia and type 2 diabetes. She denies any nausea, vomiting or diarrhoea, but on visiting the bathroom noticed dark blood in the pan.

'What are your differentials for this patient?'

Given the cardiovascular risk factors this patient has alongside a characteristic history, I would be concerned about an ischaemic event in the bowel. The patient may also be suffering from acute peptic ulcer disease, which is often epigastric in presentation and associated with nausea and vomiting. The patient may also be suffering from acute pancreatitis, though the pain tends to radiate to the back. This may also be an episode of diverticular disease which can cause PR bleeding, but tends to be left-sided pain.

'What blood investigations would you consider?'

Following resuscitation, I would request a FBC to look for signs of anaemia and leukocytosis which often accompany ischaemic bowel disease, but which may also support other differentials. U&E's would guide my fluid management of the patient and provide a renal baseline for further investigations. I would check the amylase level for signs of pancreatitis, CRP for a measure of inflammation and, importantly, perform an arterial blood gas analysis to look for a metabolic acidosis and a raised lactate level.

'How else would you investigate this patient?'

I would request a 12-lead ECG to look for signs of arrhythmias or acute cardiac events that may have caused subsequent bowel complications. I would also request an erect CXR and abdominal radiographs. The erect CXR would be to look for signs of a perforation secondary to an ischaemic bowel, although the absence of free air under the hemi-diaphragm would not rule this out. The abdominal radiograph would be to look for potential causes of bowel ischaemia such as an obstruction. Finally, I would discuss with a surgical senior and the radiologist whether to carry out a CT scan with contrast to look for evidence of ischaemia such as bowel wall thickening, dilation and thumb-printing suggestive of mucosal oedema.

'What can cause an ischaemic bowel?'

An embolism is the most common cause, which may be cardiac in origin (e.g. left-sided cardiac thrombus) or from the vasculature (e.g. atherosclerotic plaque). Blockage of the mesenteric vasculature may occur due to atherosclerosis typically at the origin of the superior mesenteric artery. The patient may also have non-occlusive causes such as shock, hypotension or cardiac failure.

'The patient's results are shown here. How would you act on these?'

Bloods:	
Hb.	10.6
WCC:	16.5
Neutrophils:	12.4
Sodium:	137

Bloods: (*Continued*)	
Potassium:	4.8
Urea:	10.5
Creatinine:	101
Amylase:	68
CRP:	120
ABG: (On air)	
pH:	7.29
PaO_2:	10.62
$PaCO_2$:	6.1
Lactate:	5.1

CT scan report summary: Bowel wall thickening, dilation and signs of submucosal oedema suggestive of ischaemic bowel.

I would immediately see the patient, and if possible, move them to the resuscitation suite, alert a suitable senior in surgery and place them nil by mouth. I would start resuscitation of the patient and assess their level of health using the ALS protocol A, B, C. Starting with the airway, I would speak with the patient and ensure there was a patent airway and no escalation was needed. I would briefly examine the chest for any gross pathologies based on inspection, palpation, percussion and auscultation of lung fields. For circulation, I would assess the fluids status of the patient by examining the skin turgor, capillary refill, tongue hydration, JVP and signs of peripheral oedema. I would gain intravenous access and review adjuncts such as oxygen saturation, ECG and blood pressure monitoring. I would examine the patient's cardiovascular system and assess her haemodynamic status based on capillary refill, presence of pallor, pulse rate, rhythm and nature and praecordium examination findings. I would begin aggressive fluid resuscitation with a Hartmann's solution and also prescribe IV antibiotics. I would react to any abnormal clinical findings and initiate therapy, at which point I would reassess the patient. Following this, I would ascertain when the patient had last eaten, if she had any medical problems, including drug allergies.

'Why would you give IV antibiotics?'

Breach and compromise of the normal mucosal barrier can cause significant migration of bacteria, further complicating an ischaemic bowel. This may be evidenced by the elevated infective and inflammatory markers. I would therefore prescribe broad-spectrum antibiotic enterics, such as a cephalosporin with metronidazole.

'What would you do after resuscitation?'

I would speak with a suitable senior in surgery and state my concerns regarding a patient with an ischaemic bowel. I would relate the relevant history, examination findings and investigation results. I would clearly state when the patient had last eaten, and which teams I had liased with (e.g. the A/E team). If permitted, I would be ready to alert the anaesthetist on-call and the theatre staff to efficiently expedite the patient for operative management.

'What operative management would this patient likely require?'

Given the results of the CT scan, suggesting ischaemic bowel changes, the patient is likely to require an immediate exploratory laparotomy, which is indicated in the presence of infarction, perforation or signs of peritonitis.

Background information

Bowel ischaemia may allude to acute mesenteric ischaemia, chronic mesenteric ichaemia or colonic ischaemia. Patients typically present with non-specific abdominal pain, which is out of proportion to the level of palpation along with any of the following presentations:

Presentation	Pathophysiology
Malaenia	Ischaemia to the bowel wall can cause sloughing of the mucosa and blood loss
Diarrhoea	Also associated with mucosal sloughing
Sitophobia	Typically, a feature of chronic ischaemia, food causes abdominal pain therefore the patient avoids food intake causing weight loss
Symptoms/signs of anaemia	This may include pallor, shortness of breath, malaise, etc.
Abdominal bruit	On examination, there may be an abdominal bruit on auscultation, suggesting vascular narrowing.

Other more advanced investigations to consider would include:

Investigation	Justification
CT scan	Usually with contrast or increasingly CT angiograms demonstrate non-specific signs of colonic ischaemia such as bowel wall thickening, dilation, mesenteric vascular blockage and mucosal oedema
Mesenteric angiography	Gold standard for diagnosing bowel ischaemia. Able to identify defects of the mesenteric vessels
Sigmoidoscopy or colonoscopy	Not suitable in the acute setting due to risk of perforation. Very useful in demonstrating signs of ischaemia and severity, including mucosal sloughing/friability. Submucosal erosions, oedema, luminal narrowing and necrosis.

Patients with evidence of infarction, perforation or peritonitis require exploratory laparotomy with potential bowel resection. In superior mesenteric artery embolus, or thrombosis, papaverine infusion with embolectomy is advocated. If embolectomy is not possible, an arterial bypass or even resection may be necessary. Papaverine infusion continues preoperatively through to the postoperative period, unless there is radiological evidence showing cessation of vasoconstriction. In thrombus situations, postoperative heparinisation is also recommended.

Clinical vignettes for further practice

A 54-year-old female complains of an intense abdominal pain that constantly occurs after she eats. She has been treated for reflux disease and has significantly reduced her portion intake. However, the pain has begun to increase in severity and led her to avoid food altogether. She suffers from hypertension and has recovered from a myocardial infarction several months ago.

Regardless of how the other stations go, keep your mind clear and focused for the clinical station, the 2 mins you spend before you go inside are crucial, spend them wisely.

2.24 KNEE PAIN

Clinical case

While holding the orthopaedic on-call bleed, you are referred a 45-year-old male farmer who has presented with a painful, swollen knee. He first noticed a mild pain and swelling in the left knee a few days ago and has tried paracetamol and ibuprofen. The knee has steadily become more painful, swollen, stiff and erythematous. He has had a farming accident in the past requiring reconstructive surgery and skin grafts of his left knee and leg which occasionally becomes stiff. He suffers from type 2 diabetes but is otherwise fit and well, and takes no regular medication other than metformin. He suffers no drug allergies and has no relevant family history. His clinical observations are:

Heart rate: 97 bpm; blood pressure: 110/80 mmHg; RR: 12; Sats: 99%.

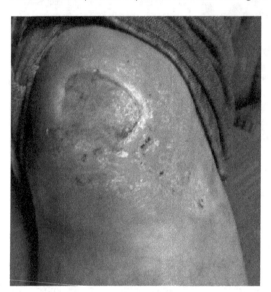

> Orthopaedic emergencies require prompt recognition and action. They are very common and often poorly managed. Learn these topics well.

'What are your differentials for this patient?'

My primary differential for this patient would be a septic arthritis of the knee, which is an orthopaedic emergency. I would also consider gout and pseudo-gout, both of which can present with a hot and swollen joint. This may also be cellulitis of the overlying skin.

'What are the risk factors for septic arthritis?'

Important risk factors would include preceding joint disease such as osteoarthritis and rheumatoid arthritis which predispose to joint infection. The presence of a joint prosthesis automatically increases the risk of developing joint sepsis. Diabetes also predisposes to increased infection risk, IV drug abusers can introduce infection, which can seed into the surrounding or even distant joints.

'What diagnostic factors would you look for in the history and examination of septic arthritis?'

I would establish the affected joint to be hot, swollen, tender and with restricted movements, which is characteristic of septic arthritis. I would also enquire if the patient was diabetic, had a history of alcoholism and/or came from a low socioeconomic background. The presence of cutaneous ulcers, prosthetic joints, underlying joint disease and previous corticosteroid injections would also be important risk factors for this pathology.

'What investigations would you consider?'

I would take a FBC, U&E, CRP and ESR. These would be useful in monitoring the progress of treatment, but are not diagnostic and do not exclude pathology. I would take blood cultures before initiating any IV antibiotics. The most helpful investigation would be a synovial joint fluid aspiration, again before starting any IV antibiotics. I would perform this under senior supervision. A radiograph of the joint would again not help in diagnosis, but would be useful for revealing any underlying joint disease such as degeneration and chondrocalcinosis.

'What investigations would you perform on the joint aspirate?'

I would first document the location, volume and description of the fluid. I would place the sample in a universal container pot and, if possible, also inoculate blood culture bottles with the sample. I would then send the aspirate for gram stain, culture, microscopy and sensitivities. The microscopic analysis may reveal the causative organisms, therefore directing antibiotic treatment. Polarising microscopy would identify the presence of urate or calcium pyrophosphate indicating gout or pseudo-gout, respectively.

'What antibiotic treatment would you prescribe?'

Gram-positive organisms are the most common causative organisms in suspected septic joints. I would review the hospital protocol first; however, empirical treatment is usually with vancomycin after joint aspiration. I would alter this treatment if gram staining and other investigation results alluded to other organisms. If the patient was allergic to vancomycin, I would consider clindamycin or a cephalosporin class of antibiotic.

Background information

A septic joint is an orthopaedic emergency and centres around the presentation of a hot, tender, swollen joint with restricted movements. The principle of investigation and treatment is joint aspiration, in all suspected cases, and the initiation of empirical treatment after aspiration and cultures have been taken.

Gram-negative infections typically affect more elderly patients and those who have had recent abdominal surgery. Empirical treatment therefore would include a third-generation cephalosporin, and – dependent on the local hospital policy – the addition of gentamicin can also be considered, assuming renal function permits this. Patients who are penicillin allergic may be given ciprofloxacin.

Intravenous drug abusers are more susceptible to pseudomonas infections for which ceftazidime is preferentially given. Treatment for all septic joints usually lasts for at least 2 weeks, followed by a further 4 weeks of oral antibiotic therapy.

Clinical vignettes for further practice

A 45-year-old female presents with a 3-day history of a hot and swollen right elbow. She suffers from osteoarthritis for which she takes NSAIDs, and has been given steroid injections on multiple occasions. Upon examination the elbow is swollen, painful on palpation and with very limited movements.

> *Try to show the interviewers that you have diagnosed, investigated and treated whatever disease they are questioning you on. Each time I was asked a question, I would say things like "I have usually treated this by..." or stating activities like checking hospital and national guidelines and policies. They don't want a fully trained surgical registrar, but they do want to see active evidence that you can become a well-trained surgical registrar.*

2.25 LEG PAIN

Clinical case

A 21-year-old male is involved in a domestic dispute while intoxicated. He presents to A/E after being stabbed in the right leg with a kitchen knife. He is brought into A/E by his friends smelling strongly of alcohol but conversant. Whilst under A/E care, he pulls the embedded knife out while awaiting review. There is no bleeding and the patient has a full complement of pulses throughout the leg which is then lightly bandaged. You are bleeped after the patient starts to complain of increasing pain and swelling in the leg an hour later, despite a normal repeated examination of the neurological and vascular system in the leg.

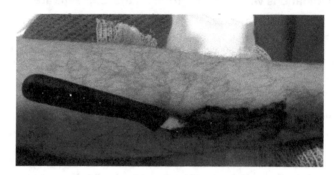

'What are your differentials for this patient?'

I would be most concerned that this patient was developing a compartment syndrome of the affected leg. Given the mechanism of injury, there may also be acute ischaemia of the limb though I would expect absent peripheral pulses. There may be a haematoma, which would be tender on palpation, with an overlying ecchymosis. The patient may also have suffered trauma or rupture of the muscles in the area of injury.

> Most candidates will memorise details, for example the cardinal symptoms and signs in compartment syndrome. You will instantly outclass them if you can show the interviewers how to use this information in the clinical setting. This can be as simple as knowing which are the most sensitive and early signs, and mentioning them first.

'What are the risk factors for developing compartment syndrome?'

Patients have most often been involved in some form of trauma. This can affect the soft tissue with or without a resultant fracture of the associated bone. Penetrating trauma can cause intra-compartmental haemorrhage and muscle oedema. External pressure through tight casts or bandages can also exert excessive compression, leading to increased compartmental pressure. Intense muscular activity over a prolonged period of time can also cause muscle swelling leading to compartment syndrome. Haemophilia sufferers and patients with external burns are also at significant risk.

'What are the cardinal symptoms and signs of compartment syndrome?'

Important symptoms of compartment syndrome would include pain, which is an early sign and often disproportionate to the injury sustained. It can be elicited with passive stretching of the muscle in the compartment that is affected. Patients may also complain of a tightness or pressure in the affected limb, which is another early indication of developing pathology. Paraesthesia is another early sign and may be in the distribution of the nerve if it travels through the affected compartment. Objective signs, which are often late, include pallor suggesting vascular insufficiency, and pulselessness, although this would need to be confirmed on doppler ultrasound. Paralysis is one of the latest signs, suggesting loss of motor function in the limb. It can be difficult to interpret as the mechanism of injury may prevent movement, however in disease pathology, prolonged nerve or muscle injury can result in permanent damage.

'How would you investigate this patient?'

If I suspected this patient to have an acute compartment syndrome, I would base my decision mostly on the clinical history and examination. Following this, I would first alert a senior in surgery before proceeding further with other investigations. If permitted, I could measure the compartment pressure using an electronic compartment measurement instrument. I would do this by inserting the probe close to the level of the injury, ideally within 5 cm, and also at multiple sites of the compartment. I could also measure the serum creatine kinase, which would indicate muscle necrosis for which renal function monitoring would be important.

'Would you use the compartment pressure itself to direct your management?'

No. I would ideally calculate the differential pressure in the compartment. I would do this by subtracting the measured compartment pressure from the diastolic blood pressure, assuming the patient was not on vasodilatory cardiac medications. If the differential pressure was <20 mmHg, this would strongly indicate compartment syndrome and indicate a fasciotomy.

'What supportive treatments would you initiate while awaiting senior review?'

I would remove any dressings and bandages from the affected limb; if there was a cast, I would split this completely and ensure the circumference of the limb was completely free. I would then prescribe patient-controlled opiate-based analgesic, assuming they were not allergic to this. I would also prescribe and initiate a fluid infusion ensuring the patient maintains a urine output >35 mLs/hour to protect the kidneys from the effects of rhabdomyolysis. Finally, I would elevate the leg to at least the level of the heart with regular neurovascular review.

Background information

Compartment syndrome of a limb describes the microvascular compromise of a closed compartment due to restricted capillary blood flow. The most commonly affected of these include the anterior and deep leg compartments and the volar compartment of the forearm. The compartment is at significant risk of damage if the compartment pressure is within 10–30 mmHg of the patients' diastolic blood pressure, or if the absolute pressure exceeds 30–40 mmHg, although this is not always accurate.

Compartment syndrome may be classed as acute or chronic. Acute pathology is most often due to direct trauma to the bone or soft tissue, leading to oedema and haemorrhage with subsequent increase in the interstitial compartment pressure. Chronic compartment syndrome describes a pathology most often seen in athletes who undertake intense muscular activity with recurrent episodes of pain.

If supportive therapy fails, a fasciotomy of all compartments with increased pressures is indicated, ideally within 6 hours of the start of pressure increase. The viability of muscle can be reviewed in the theatre, and postoperatively meticulous wound care is needed to prevent infection. Patients suffering from compartment syndrome >8 hours after its onset, alongside a compromised muscle function, may be eligible for a primary amputation, even if the neurological function is intact.

Clinical vignettes for further practice

A 45-year-old male presents to A/E after suffering from a motorcycle incident. He is found to have a displaced distal tibia and fibula fracture of the right leg, which is successfully reduced and placed in a cast. The following day he complains of increased pain and tightness in the affected leg despite receiving adequate analgesic. The cast is split and on examination the limb is neurologically intact, however you notice the right leg is considerably paler compared to the left despite normal pulses in both legs.

> " Treat the scenario as realistically as possible. I was just finishing a rotation in general surgery and felt quite comfortable with the basic general surgery questions but stumbled at the very beginning. The examiner said a nurse had called me to review a patient, I immediately launched into resuscitating and was stopped by the interviewer who said that you are on the phone. These basic things like listening carefully, and using your experience of real situations, really count and matter so don't overlook them. "

2.26 LIMPING CHILD

Clinical case

You are asked to see a 15-year-old male who has been limping due to a right-sided hip and knee pain. He denies any preceding trauma. He did visit his GP yesterday who stated he was likely suffering from growing pains from pubertal changes. Upon examination, the child has a large body habitus, and when examining his gait, it is discovered that he leans over to the right side. On examination, there is no pain on palpation of the right knee which also has a good range of movement. The leg, however, sits in an externally rotated position.

'What could this patient be suffering from?'

In this age group the patient may be suffering from a slipped capital femoral epiphysis which often affects children during puberty, particularly if they are overweight. Although usually in a younger group of patients this may also be Perthes' disease, which can present in a very similar fashion. There has been no preceding trauma, however the patient may have suffered a simple groin pull or muscular injury. This would typically present with pain on adduction, but I would not expect the leg to be in an external rotation. Finally, I would also consider the possibility of a stress fracture.

'What diagnostic investigation would you request?'

I would request bilateral AP radiographs of the hips. This would be to diagnose the presence of a slipped capital femoral epiphysis, as well as rule out other differentials. I would look to see if Klein's line intersects through the femoral head. For a more sensitive view, I would request a frog lateral radiograph and again examine for a normal Klein's line and the Bloomberg's sign. It would be good practice to get a radiograph of the knee to ensure no abnormality existed, and to consider lumbar radiographs also.

You will not be expected to report anything but the very basic operative orthopaedic management, for example the principles of open reduction and internal fixation. We have included more detail here for your clinical acumen and to set you apart from other candidates.

'What are Klein's lines and the Bloomberg sign?'

This is a line that is drawn along the superior border of the femoral neck, in normal patients this line with pass through a portion of the femoral head. In a slipped metaphysis, the line will miss the femoral head. The Bloomberg sign can be interpreted on a frog lateral radiograph and shows widening or blurring of the physis.

Klein's line in a normal and slipped diagram

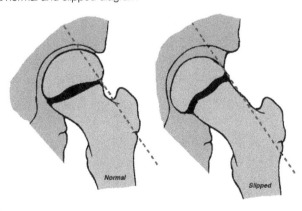

Normal   Slipped

'How do patients with a slipped capital femoral epiphysis usually present?'

Patients usually have hip pain, however, this may be referred to the groin or knee. Hip pain can often be bilateral and associated with reduced movements at the hip, particularly flexion. Upon examination, the patient may exhibit a Trendelenburg gait whereby on walking they lean toward the affected side. Active and passive flexion movements of the hip are likely to be limited and may also cause pain.

'What is the treatment of an unstable slipped capital femoral epiphysis?'

The patient would require urgent surgical repair which would involve decompressing the hip joint, and reducing the slipped segment followed by screw fixation. The contralateral hip may also be fixed, though this is often at the discretion of the operating consultant.

Background information

Previously known as slipped upper femoral epiphysis, this still remains a misnomer. In a slipped capital femoral epiphysis, it is the metaphysis that is displaced. The abnormality typically affects adolescents and the cause is often idiopathic, however, there are important risk factors associated. These include puberal growth, obesity and particular endocrine disorders such as hypothyroidism, panhypopituitarism, renal osteodystrophy and growth hormone deficiency. The aetiology is thought to be due to raised stress factors causing shearing at the growth plate, which results in weakening and widening of the physis. Following repair, patients should be followed up at 2 weeks for a wound review as well as a functional assessment, including the ability to walk and a radiographic assessment.

Clinical vignettes for further practice

A 13-year-old female suffers a fall at school onto her left side while running, 3 days later she complains of pain in her right hip and has been unable to fully bear weight on this side. She also mentions being bullied at school due to recent gains in weight. Upon examination, there is no bruising or pain in the left leg, however, the right hip has restricted movements.

> *I was dreading orthopaedics coming up in my station, but the questions are all logical and based on principles. Don't waste your time learning any in-depth operations. Knowing the foundations really well will hold you in good stead.*

2.27 NECK LUMP

Clinical case

You are referred a 34-year-old female who has presented with a neck lump. She complains of a tightness at the neck and constantly sweating regardless of the room temperature. She has suffered significant weight loss despite an increase in appetite and constantly feels jittery. She has no difficulty in breathing and feels no pain at her neck, but has felt an increasingly large lump. Upon examination, a smooth right-sided neck mass is palpable; there is no exophthalmos or pretibial myxoedema, but a mild lid lag is present. Her observations are:

Heart rate: 105; blood pressure: 150/85 mmHg; RR: 18.

'What are your differentials?'

This patient appears to be suffering from the consequences of hyperthyroidism. The finding of a single enlarged nodule suggests this may be a toxic thyroid adenoma. This may also be Graves' disease, though exopthalmos and pretibial myxoedema are usually present. On examination, only a single nodule was palpable, but this may also be a toxic multinodular goitre.

> The clinical vignette is usually directive with regards to the diagnosis. However, this can sometimes be more elusive allowing a broader discussion based on your differentials. The interviewers may help you if you miss an important pathology, or steer the discussion in a different direction.

'What is the pathophysiology of a toxic thyroid adenoma?'

This is a benign malignancy of the thyroid that is outside of the control of the thyroid stimulating hormone. The tumour produces thyroid hormones at levels which are inappropriately elevated compared to the level required by the body, resulting in symptoms and signs of hyperthyroidism.

'What diagnostic symptoms and signs would you expect? '

I would expect the patient to complain of a number of characteristic changes relating to a state of hyperthyroidism. These include hyperphagia alongside a concurrent unintentional loss in weight, and feelings of

> Lid lag is commonly present across multiple hyperthyroid pathologies. It can be suggestive of Graves' disease but is not a cardinal sign, unlike exopthalmos or pretibial myxoedema.

nervousness or anxiety. Objective signs may include increased defaecation, oligomenorrhoea, warm moist skin and tachycardia. I would not expect to see signs of Graves' disease including exopthalmos and pretibial myxoedema.

'What specific investigations would you consider in this patient?'

Following resuscitation among other investigations, I would request TSH level, free T4, and total T3. I would expect the TSH level to be suppressed as a diagnostic feature of thyroid abnormality. I would also expect the T4 level to be raised, although the T3 level is more helpful and reliable since in subclinical hyperthyroidism T4 levels can be normal. I would also request an ECG to look for signs of dysrhythmias. A thyroid scan would be diagnostic, as it would demonstrate a 'hot nodule' from iodine isotope uptake. I would consider a CT scan if there were any signs of neck compression, or as part of a preoperative planning.

'What investigations could help you differentiate between Graves' disease and toxic adenoma?'

If I was equivocal regarding the diagnosis between Graves' disease and toxic adenoma, I would request thyroid peroxidase antibodies, which are sensitive for Graves' disease. A TSH hormone receptor antibodies test is also helpful, particularly if a patient cannot undergo a nuclear scan, such as during pregnancy. Antimicrosomal antibodies are relatively sensitive in Graves' disease but can also indicate another pathology such as Hashimoto's disease. A thyroid ultrasound scan may be useful if a thyroid isotope scan was cold in the region of a palpable nodule when diagnosing toxic thyroid adenoma.

'How would you manage this patient if investigations confirm toxic thyroid adenoma?'

Although this patient is relatively stable, I would consider first gaining medical control with antithyroid medication such as thiamazole, which inhibits thyroperoxidase. I would ensure the patient was not pregnant or lactating, and offer radioactive iodine therapy. Symptoms may also require beta blockade if severe. Antithyroid treatment would be stopped shortly before radioactive treatment and restarted 3–5 days afterward. More definitive treatment would involve a subtotal thyroidectomy, which avoids radioactivity and gains thyroid control more quickly. I would involve the patient in making these decisions.

'If the patient was pregnant or lactating what would be your first line management?'

I would advise thiamazole except in the first trimester of pregnancy. Although propylthiouracil works by the same mechanism, it has a higher risk of hepatotoxicity, but in the first trimester thiamazole is associated with congenital defects.

Background information

The assessment of a thyroid mass centres on differentiating a benign lesion from a more sinister or dangerous one. Important risk factors or presentations you should be aware of include:

- Rapidly enlarging neck mass: This can lead to airway compromise and patients may present with a stridor or hoarseness. This can occur in anaplastic thyroid cancer, or haemorrhage into a nodule of a thyroid adenoma
- Incidental neck masses should not be ignored and triple assessment with history/examination, ultrasound scanning and fine needle aspiration, based on imaging results, should be undertaken to determine the nature of the disease
- Iodine deficiency: This is the commonest cause for nodular goitre formation

Head and neck irradiation, such as in lymphoma treatment, can also be a risk factor for thyroid malignancy.

Interpreting thyroid function tests:

Disease	TSH	fT4	Ft3
Iodine induced hyperthyroidism	↓	↑	↑
Toxic thyroid adenoma	↓	↑	↑
Toxic multinodular goitre	↓	↑	↑
Graves' disease	↓	↑	↑
Hashimoto's thyroiditis	↑	↓	↓
Irradiation	↑	↓	↓
Thyroidectomy	↑	↓	↓

Clinical vignettes for further practice

A 32-year-old female complains of increasingly blurred vision. She has recently been promoted at work and attributes her weight loss and feelings of anxiety to stress. She frequently experiences palpitations and has noticed changes in the appearance of her eyes. She has finally become concerned after noticed a growing mass at the centre of her neck.

> *In hindsight, I didn't take my interview seriously enough. I had read general surgery topics and had completed almost 12 months of general surgery rotations. I had good experience in theatre but the interviewers ask questions that can easily determine if you have been around the wards with patients. My friends had far less experience than me but practised scenarios properly along with some reading. Not surprisingly they received offers while I didn't.*

2.28 NECK OF FEMUR FRACTURE

Clinical case

You are referred a 65-year-old female who has suffered a fall whilst trying to get out of bed. She landed on her right side and was unable to mobilise back to her feet without the aid of her husband. She denies any preceding dizziness, shortness of breath or chest pain. She has pain in her right hip and is unable to bear weight. On examination, the right leg is shortened and externally rotated, the neurological and vascular status of the leg is intact, and there are no other injuries. She suffers from hypertension, asthma and osteoporosis.

'How would you proceed with this patient?'

I would begin by resuscitating the patient and assess her level of health using the ALS protocol A, B, C. Starting with the airway, I would speak with the patient and ensure there was a patent airway and no escalation was needed. I would briefly examine the chest for any gross pathologies based on inspection, palpation, percussion and auscultation of the lung fields. For circulation, I would assess the fluids status of the patient by examining the skin turgor, capillary refill, tongue hydration, JVP and signs of peripheral oedema. I would gain intravenous access, send for routine bloods and review appropriate adjuncts such as the oxygen saturation, ECG monitoring and blood pressure monitoring. I would examine the patient's cardiovascular system and assess her haemodynamic status based on capillary refill, presence of pallor, pulse rate, rhythm and nature and praecordium examination findings. I would react to any abnormal clinical findings and initiate therapy, at which point I would reassess the patient. Once the patient is stable, I would then take a focused history based on the patient's presenting complaint and relevant past medical and drug history, as well as social circumstances.

'What is the likely diagnosis in this patient?'

Given the mechanism of injury and the patient's inability to mobilise or bear weight alongside the deformity of the right leg, I would be most concerned about a right neck of femur fracture. I would also wish to ensure there were no other bony fractures, as well as ensure there are no precipitants to the fall.

> A shortened and externally rotated leg is commonly associated with a neck of femur fracture. However, you should also ensure there is no pelvic, femoral shaft or tibia fracture.

'What important risk factors are associated with neck of femur fractures?'

The mechanism of injury – usually falls from a height in the elderly, or high energy trauma such as road traffic accidents in the young, are strongly associated with sustaining a proximal femoral fracture. The presence of osteoporosis, or osteopaenia, poses a significant risk to sustaining proximal femoral fractures, alongside increasing age. Females are also more likely to suffer from a neck of femur fracture, and this may in part be related to the onset of menopause.

'How would you classify hip fractures?'

Hip fractures extend from the head of the femur to just below the lesser trochanter, and may be classified in relation to the hip joint capsule being intra-capsular or extra-capsular. Intracapsular fractures may be below the head of the femur (subcapital), across the mid-femoral neck (transcervical) or across the base of the femoral neck (basicervical). Extracapsular fractures are outside the hip capsule and include intertrochanteric and subtrochanteric fractures. Strictly speaking, extra-capsular fractures do qualify as neck of femur fractures.

'How would you classify neck of femur fractures?'

I would use the Garden's classification for fractures of the femoral neck, of which there are four types. Type 1 fractures are incomplete or impacted with valgus angulation of the distal fragment. Type 2 involve fractures that traverse the entire neck, but remain undisplaced. Type 3 is a partially displaced fracture that runs across the whole neck of the femur, whilst type 4 fractures traverse the entire neck and are completely displaced.

'How would you investigate this patient?'

Following resuscitation, I would request a urine dipstick primarily to look for signs of a urinary tract infection, I would request an FBC again to look for signs of infection which may have precipitated a fall. I would review the U&Es to establish a baseline of renal function, which would be important when considering further investigations and also possible operative management. I would include a crossmatch of 2 units and a coagulation screen as preparation for theatre. An ECG would be important to again check for any signs of cardiovascular distress such as arrhythmias, which may explain a non-mechanical fall. This would also be important from an anaesthetic view point, if operative management is planned. For orthopaedic management, I would request an AP and lateral view of the affected hip. An internal rotation view of the hip, whereby the hip is rotated internally by 15 degrees, would also be helpful to show fractures of the proximal femur.

'What would you do if the radiographs showed no fracture, but the patient remained in pain?'

I would consider requesting an MRI scan that may show evidence of a marrow oedema and an occult fracture line, which is easily missed on a radiograph. If an MRI was unavailable or unsuitable, I would then consider a CT scan, which again may reveal an occult fracture.

'What would be the management of an undisplaced fracture in this patient?'

The ideal management would be an internal fixation of the fracture using a dynamic hip screw, or multiple cannulated screws alongside prophylactic antibiotics.

Background information

This is an extremely common occurrence amongst the elderly, most of whom suffer low energy or low impact mechanical falls. Age and osteoporosis are common denominating factors. Patients typically present with an inability to bear weight, particularly in displaced fractures of the hip. Movement of the hip is generally restricted with pain exacerbation on hip flexion, as well as on internal and external rotation. The hip is classically shortened and externally rotated, typically due to muscle action such as when the adductor muscle spasms following injury. Important differential diagnoses to consider include:

Differential	Description	Investigation
Femoral head fracture	Usually associated with hip dislocation	Usually diagnosed on radiograph or CT scan
Femoral shaft fracture	Associated with thigh deformity	Diagnosed on radiograph
Acetabular fracture	Leg shortening and external rotation is not usually a feature	Usually diagnosed on radiograph
Sepsis	May involve prolonged injury, fever and rigors	Serum investigation and joint aspirate
Pubic rami fracture	Leg shortening and external rotation is not usually a feature	Usually diagnosed on radiograph or MRI

In displaced fractures, internal fixation is generally advocated for patients <60 years old to avoid avascular necrosis. Fracture fixation is usually at the discretion of the operating consultant when opting for dynamic hip screw, or the use of multiple screws for fixation. Beyond the age of 60, treatment options may encompass internal fixation or arthroplasty with debatable evidence at present. In all patients, the use of prophylactic antibiotics, postoperative pain relief and physiotherapy is strongly recommended.

Clinical vignettes for further practice

An 82-year-old male is brought into A/E after suffering a fall while walking. He normally uses a walking stick to mobilise and recalls feeling disorientated before tripping over a curb. He has suffered a myocardial infarction in the past and is on medication for hypertension and diabetes. Upon examination, the left leg is shortened and externally rotated with bruising of the left trochanter.

> *You will develop a rhythm as you practise scenarios more and more. It can seem repetitive at first but each surgical disease has a particular emphasis, e.g. the optimisation of an elderly patient with a fracture or the resuscitation of a patient with an aortic aneurysm. Put in the practice, and it will pay dividends.*

2.29 OESOPHAGEAL PERFORATION

Clinical case

You are referred a 39-year-old female who complains of severe chest pains following a bout of binge drinking. After vomiting food on multiple occasions, she fell asleep at a friends' house but awoke feeling shortness of breath and severe retrosternal chest pain. She admits to suffering from recently diagnosed bulimia and has had oesophageal reflux symptoms in the past, but states her current pain is much worse. An ECG is normal and the following observations are recorded:

Heart rate: 107; blood pressure: 133/92 mmHg; RR: 22; Sats: 94%: Temp: 38.3.

'What are your differentials for this patient?'

My primary diagnosis for this patient would be an oesophageal perforation given the preceding history of vomiting and characteristic symptoms, and this would be a surgical emergency. The patient may also have a Mallory–Weiss tear, although this tends to present with haematemesis and mild chest pain. The patient may also be suffering from gastro-oesophageal reflux disease, which can present with chest pain and shortness of breath.

> Mallory–Weiss tears and oesophageal perforation are similar conditions that share risk factors. The former is much less severe having weak associations with hiatus hernia and NSAID use.

'What are the characteristic features of an oesophageal perforation?'

Patients typically present following heavy drinking or eating episodes, with some form of forceful action such as vomiting. Retrosternal or upper abdominal pain and shortness of breath are most often associated, although the patient may also complain of odynophagia and shoulder pain. Examination findings are usually limited but subcutaneous emphysema is an important associated finding. Auscultation may also reveal a crunching sound synchronous with the heart beat, known as Hamman's sign. The triad of chest pain, vomiting and subcutaneous emphysema is known as Mackler's triad.

'Once stabilised what investigations would you consider?'

I would request an FBC and CRP for signs of infection, and estimate the degree of inflammation and sepsis that may have occurred. I would review the U&Es to guide fluid resuscitation and replace losses incurred from vomiting. A chest radiograph would be important to look for signs of a pleural effusion, most of which are left sided, and a pneumomediastinum. The most diagnostic investigation would be a water-soluble contrast such as gastrograffin. A CT scan can be performed in a stable patient for further diagnostics, but may also identify precipitants to the rupture such as malignancy or fistula formation.

'Why would you use a water-soluble contrast medium rather than barium contrast?'

A water soluble contrast has high sensitivity for diagnosing an oesophageal rupture, and if there is a large leak, extravasation causes much less irritation to the mediastinum than a barium contrast. The gastrograffin is given to the patient whilst lying in the right lateral decubitus position to provide the most accurate results.

'What is the definitive management for this patient?'

Management may be operative or non-operative. Conservative treatment aims to limit the degree of mediastinitis and appropriate in situations such as iatrogenic perforation e.g.

endoscopy. In this patient, who has signs of sepsis, a direct primary repair of the oesophagus can be attempted. In the presence of an abscess, drainage or an external fistula can be created. In severe cases, oesophageal resection may be required.

Background information

The most common causes of an oesophageal perforation are iatrogenic such as during an endoscopy, or as a consequence of barotrauma or Boerhaave's syndrome. The latter classically occurs on vomiting against a close glottis, with subsequent rupture. Patients typically present with severe chest pain, upper abdominal pain and shortness of breath at the time of injury. Subcutaneous emphysema may occur approximately 1 hour after the injury. Severe sepsis and mediastinitis can occur as early as 4 hours after injury. Conservative operative management may be guided by review of the following areas:

- Perforation site (thoracoabdominal usually more severe than cervical)
- Aetiology (spontaneous vs. instrumental)
- Underlying (benign or malignant)
- Food presence in the oesophagus prior to perforation

Direct primary repair is ideally performed in the first 4–6 hours after which the tissues become more inflammed, swollen and friable. Late presenting patients are more often managed with an external fistula. This can be achieved through the insertion of a T-tube with drain insertion to allow removal of extravasated material. Oesophagectomy is reserved for the most severe cases, for example when there is evidence of necrosis.

Clinical vignettes for further practice

A 45-year-old male is referred directly to surgical care after undergoing an endoscopy for dyspeptic symptoms. The registrar performing the investigation noticed a large mass in the distal part of the oesophagus, but caused an accidental perforation whilst examining it. The patient is relatively stable and pain free at present but complains of severe chest pain.

> Don't focus your efforts all in one area. The year I applied all of the stations had an equal weighting, but I found myself spending most of my time in the clinical section. Excelling in one station is not enough to compensate for a poor performance in any of the other stations.

2.30 PAINFUL TESTIS

Clinical case

You are a referred an 8-year-old male child who awoke with acute pain in the right testis. The child appears in considerable discomfort and affirms feeling nauseated and has vomited whilst in the department. Upon examination there is a tender, swollen right testicle, which is painful on palpation. He also has mild tenderness on palpation of the suprapubic region. He is apyrexial and observations are within normal limits.

'What are your differentials for this patient?'

My primary diagnosis for this patient would be a testicular torsion which is a surgical emergency, and one that I would wish to investigate and act on immediately. My differentials would include epididymitis, although I would expect this to have a more prolonged presentation over a few days, rather than an acute presentation. Epididymo-orchitis would also similarly present over a few days, and may also have fever and urinary symptoms alongside it. I would also consider a torsion of a testicular appendage though this often presents with localised superior testicle pain, and is not typically associated with nausea or vomiting. Finally, I would also wish to exclude an acute appendicitis though this would not usually cause concomitant testicular swelling.

'What are the classical features of a testicular torsion?'

Patients typically complain of severe testicular pain, which may be relapsing and remitting, but often occurs abruptly. This is usually accompanied by nausea and vomiting. Patients may also less frequently complain of accompanying abdominal pain, fever and urinary frequency. Upon examination, there may be scrotal swelling and erythema,

> Knowing the classical examination findings for surgical diseases helps to support the primary diagnosis. Make it clear to the interviewer which signs you place more weight upon, and others that are more supplementary.

palpation is often exquisitely tender and there is no relief on elevating the scrotum. I would specifically look for a high-riding testicle, which would be elevated and may also have a horizontal lie compared to its normal, unaffected counterpart. Finally, I would examine for the cremasteric reflex, which is often absent in testicular torsion.

'What risk factors do you know of that contribute to testicular torsion?'

Important risk factors in testicular torsion would include male patients aged between 12–18 years old, as the incidence of testicular torsion is higher in this group, although males of any age can suffer from this condition. Patients with a bell clapper deformity are also at a higher risk of suffering a testicular torsion, since the testicle can rotate freely within the tunica vaginalis and in doing so cause a torsion. An undescended testis also has a much higher incidence of torsion. Although less important, I would also be aware of a preceding trauma to the genital area that can cause a torsion, and episodes of intermittent pain in the past, which can represent a twisting and untwisting testicular pedicle.

'How would you treat this patient?'

Following resuscitation, I would alert my senior in surgery and ideally seek urological advice. I would state that I was worried the patient might have a testicular torsion. I would give the patient analgesic, which would help reduce his pain and anxiety, making future examinations easier. Treatment may involve manual detorsion whilst preparations are made in theatre. Under supervision, I would do this by gently rotating the affected testicle, as if opening a book. The aim would be to provide temporary relief before definitive treatment, which would be scrotal exploration.

Background information

Testicular torsion represents a urological emergency resulting from the twisting of the testicle upon its spermatic cord, compromising the vascular supply with a resultant tissue ischaemia. You should always have a high index of suspicion in such patients and a low threshold for escalation.

There is a bimodal distribution of incidence primarily affecting neonates and adolescents. Testicular torsion can be classified as intra-vaginal, extra-vaginal and secondary to a long mesorchium. Intra-vaginal torsion is the most common type, resulting from an abnormally high attachment of the tunica vaginalis to the spermatic cord. This permits movement of the testicle in a rotational manner with a risk of torsion. Extra-vaginal torsion is a rarer cause, occurring due to testicle descent with twisting around the spermatic cord. The mesorchium is a band of connective tissue that attaches the epididymus to the posterolateral testis wall. A long mesorchium may allow rotational movement of the testis, which may again permit torsion.

Differential	Important features
Testicular appendage torsion	More gradual pain onset typically without nausea or vomiting, with normal cremasteric reflexes The 'blue dot sign', a blue dot visible through the scrotal skin represents the torted appendage
Epididymitis or epididymo-orchitis	Gradual onset infero-posterior testicular pain associated with urinary frequency and dysuria. Urine analysis is often abnormal
Testicular cancer	Pain may or may not be a feature with incidental mass detection. May be accompanied by enlarged lymphadenopathy
Inguinal hernia	May present with a mass in the inguinal canal that proceeds into the scrotum. The scrotum typically has a normal lie and reflexes, and is not usually painful.

Clinical vignettes for further practice

A 14-year-old male presents to A/E complaining of increasingly severe left testicular pain. He noticed the pain soon after playing football and thought it was muscle pain. He has felt nauseated but has not vomited. Upon examination, the left testicle is swollen and erythematous and too painful to palpate.

> Try to keep as calm and professional as possible during the interview. I lost my train of thought a few times because the interviewer interrupted my answer and asked another question. My other friends mentioned a similar thing during their interviews, and this is more the interviewer being satisfied and wanting to move on, but it can knock your momentum when you're in the station.

2.31 PERFORATION

Clinical case

A 64-year-old male attends A/E while you are on-call. The A/E registrar is concerned that the patient looks unwell and moves him to the resuscitation bay and asks for your help. The patient complains of a 5-day history of increasing abdominal pain, nausea, vomiting and generally feeling unwell. He suffers from well-controlled hypertension, but is otherwise well and has no relevant surgical history. Upon examination, the patient has a large body habitus, and there is generalised pain that is most acute in the left lower quadrant of the patient. His abdomen feels rigid despite your requests to ask the patient to relax. No masses are palpable. His observations are:

Heart rate: 120; blood pressure: 89/62 mmHg; RR: 16; Sats: 96% on air; Temp: 38.8.

'What do you think is happening to this patient?'

This appears to be a clinically unstable patient who has no obvious past medical or surgical history, but is suffering from an acute abdomen. He appears to be peritonitic with pain diffusely present, although more pronounced in the left iliac fossa. My differentials for this patient would include a perforated viscus such as diverticulitis, appendicitis or peptic ulcer. I would also consider other abnormalities such as a mesenteric ischaemia, pancreatitis and an abdominal aortic aneurysm.

> Be ready when a sick patient is presented to you. These vignettes or topics of discussion will separate those candidates that are safe and worth considering. Do not become complacent and overlook basic principles such as resuscitation. Showing the interviewer you can safely support a sick patient is much more relevant and helpful than knowing advanced surgical details.

'How would you proceed with this patient?'

I would alert a surgical senior and proceed with resuscitation of the patient and assess their level of health using the ALS protocol A, B, C. Starting with airway, I would speak with the patient and ensure there was a patent airway and no escalation was needed. I would briefly examine the chest for any gross pathologies based on inspection, palpation, percussion and auscultation of lung fields. For circulation, I would assess the fluid status of the patient by examining the skin turgor, capillary refill, tongue hydration, JVP and signs of peripheral oedema. I would gain intravenous access and review adjuncts such as oxygen saturation, ECG monitoring and blood pressure monitoring. I would request a full set of bloods for any pathology including FBC, U&E, LFTs, clotting and cross match for 4 units of blood and an ABG to review acid-base status, oxygenation and lactate levels. I would examine the patient's cardiovascular system and assess his haemodynamic status based on capillary refill, presence of pallor, pulse rate, rhythm and nature and praecordium examination findings. I would react to any abnormal clinical findings and initiate therapy, at which point I would reassess the patient.

'What single diagnostic investigation would you request and why?'

In order to confirm my diagnosis I would request a CT scan of the abdomen with contrast if renal function permits, once the patient was in a more stable condition. Although an erect CXR is a helpful first-line investigation, it is not diagnostic. CT imaging is reliable and accurate in identifying intra-abdominal abscesses or foreign materials. An US scan would be helpful when transport of the patient is difficult but is operator dependent and, therefore, more likely to miss a pathology. Also, patient factors such as body habitus and position of intra-abdominal organs can also contribute to false results.

'How would you interpret this CT scan?'

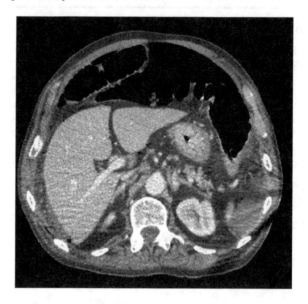

There is a large pneumoperitoneum, as noted on the erect chest radiograph. The wall of the hepatic flexure of the colon is markedly thickened in keeping with the presence of a tumour. This is taken to be the site of perforation, and supported by a preponderance of free fluid and gas around this area, extending around the liver. There is upstream dilatation of the ascending colon, and marked dilatation of the small bowel. I cannot see any obvious abnormalities of the other abdominal organs such as the liver, gallbladder and pancreas.

'How would you act on this result. Which teams would you contact?'

Although the scan result appears to show a large pneumoperitoneum, I do not feel comfortable in interpreting CT scan images. I would first review the patient again and see if they were stable and responding to the therapy that was initiated. Following this, I would then speak to the consultant radiologist and ask their advice in interpreting the CT scan. On receiving a formal report or verbal confirmation, I would record the date, time and conversation in the notes, and inform the consultant on-call.

'The consultant wishes to operate on the patient and asks you to make preparations for theatre. Which groups of people would you speak to?'

If plans were made for operative management, and assuming the patient was nil by mouth and resuscitated as before, I would confirm with the consultant they were happy for me to undertake the following actions. I would inform the anaesthetist on-call and present this patient, including relevant results. I would inform the A/E senior and nursing staff that the patient was headed for the theatre, and to allow for the necessary preparations for safe transfer. I would then proceed to the theatre and inform the site manager and theatre nurse in charge about the patient and the operation being proposed. Finally, I would make arrangements for the family to be notified and attend the hospital, although it would be preferable for the consultant to speak to them directly.

Background information

Viscus perforation results in an intra-abdominal abscess formation which causes peritonitis with high mortality. The most common causes include complications due to appendicitis, diverticulitis or surgical interventions. Causes can be classified as outlined here:

Location	Aetiology
Subphrenic, right iliac fossa, left iliac fossa, paracolic areas, pelvic	Perforation of viscus e.g. appendicitis, diverticulitis, peptic ulcer, inflammatory bowel disease, carcinoma.
Retroperitoneal	
Pancreatic, renal	Pancreatitis, pyelonephritis
Visceral	
Hepatic, splenic	Ascending cholangitis, trauma

Dependent on the cause, operative management of a perforation may follow the stepwise approach listed in the following:

- In a contained abscess, a CT or ultrasound guided drainage may be organised, e.g., appendiceal perforation and abscess formation. This is often not suitable for uncontrolled perforations, e.g., anastomotic leak, transcavity involvement, etc.
- Surgical drainage via laparotomy is performed for large events such as anastomotic leaks or where drainage is complicated or not viable. In advanced disease multi-step operations may need to be planned.
- In both situations the prescription of intravenous antibiotics should be started at the moment sepsis is recognised. This usually involves broad spectrum antibiotics, e.g. meropenem, tazobactam, etc.

Clinical vignettes for further practice

A 29-year-old female presents to A/E with nausea, vomiting, central abdominal pain which moved to the right iliac fossa and diarrhoea. She suffered the symptoms soon after eating at a takeaway shop and was diagnosed with food poisoning and discharged home. 5 days later she presents to A/E acutely unwell and septic. She was found collapsed at home and on examination has fever, hypotension, tachycardia and a rigid abdomen with signs of peritonism.

> *During your preparation for the interviews you will hear horror stories of having images and results to interpret. Although this is daunting, a good practice to get into is not to automatically refer to the official report of an investigation but look at the images and try to interpret them. Rather than just attending theatre, learn the processes involved in transporting a patient from the ward down to the theatres and note the teams involved from the porters to the consultants. Showing the interviewers that you are organised and proactive served me much better than the hours I spent re-learning clinical material although that also has a part to play. Everyone will learn how to diagnose and treat appendicitis, the best learn the clinical, administrative and logistical factors that are involved also.*

2.32 POSTOPERATIVE COUGH

Clinical case

You are bleeped by the nursing staff regarding a 45-year-old male who is recovering from a laparoscopic cholecystectomy performed 2 days ago. He has been complaining of shortness of breath and producing moderate volumes of clear phlegm, but denies any chest pain. Reviewing his observation charts, you note he has become pyrexial but is otherwise stable. He suffers from hyperlipidaemia, obesity and COPD. He is a previously heavy smoker.

'How would you proceed with this patient?'

I would resuscitate the patient and assess their level of health using the ALS protocol A, B, C. Starting with the airway I would speak with the patient and ensure there was a patent airway and no escalation was needed. I would briefly examine the chest for any gross pathologies based on inspection, palpation, percussion and auscultation of the lung fields. For circulation, I would asses the fluids status

> Commonly asked questions are often based on presentations on the ward as well as during an on-call. Be familiar with common postoperative complications and their management.

of the patient by examining the skin turgor, capillary refill, tongue hydration, JVP and signs of peripheral oedema. I would gain intravenous access, oxygen saturation and review monitoring adjuncts such as pulse oximetry, blood pressure, and an ECG. I would request a routine set of bloods including an ABG to review acid-base status, oxygenation and lactate levels. I would examine the patient's cardiovascular system and assess their haemodynamic status based on capillary refill, presence of pallor, pulse rate, rhythm and nature and praecordium examination findings. I would react to any abnormal clinical findings and initiate therapy, at which point I would reassess the patient. Once the patient is stable, I would then take a focused history based on the patient's presenting complaint and relevant past medical and drug history, as well as social circumstances.

'What are your differentials for this patient?'

My primary diagnosis for this patient suffering from shortness of breath and pyrexia shortly after an operative intervention is atelectasis. I would also consider other related abnormalities including ventilator-associated pneumonia, aspiration pneumonia and pulmonary embolism. I would also check other access sites that may have become infected such as catheters, the central venous line and cannulas.

'How would you exclude a pulmonary embolism in this patient?'

I would examine the result of the arterial blood gas and look for favourable PaO_2 and $PaCO_2$ values, or more specifically, an alveolar-arterial gradient less than 20 mmHg. I would examine the ECG recording and look for signs of a pulmonary embolism such as tachycardia, new presentations of right axis deviation and right bundle branch block. There may also be the characteristic finding of an S-wave in lead 1 and Q-waves with T-wave inversion in lead 3. I would combine these investigations along with my clinical suspicion to produce a risk score, using a suitable scoring system such as the Wells score, PERC score or the Geneva score. A chest radiograph would also be helpful for the primary diagnosis and a pulmonary embolism.

'How would a chest radiograph help you differentiate between atelectasis and a pulmonary embolism?'

I would look for signs suggestive of atelectasis, which may vary depending on the type of atelectasis. These would include increased opacification of an airless segment of lung, narrowing of intercostal spaces, compensatory hyper-expansion and displacement of fissures. Pulmonary embolism signs may include a prominent central pulmonary artery (Fleischner's sign), an elevated hemidiaphragm and a reduced perfusion in the area of the embolism (Westermark's sign).

'What are the risk factors in this patient that may cause atelectasis?'

This patients' pre-existing lung disease, alongside his previous heavy smoking, are strong risk factors that will result in excessive mucus production and a reduced ability to adequately remove these from the tracheobronchial tree. Other factors, such as laparoscopic surgery, can cause splinting of the diaphragm secondary to carbon dioxide insufflation with reduced ventilation of the lung bases and contributing to alveoli collapse. Finally, obesity and reduced mobilisation following the procedure further contribute to reduced clearance of lung secretions.

'How would you treat this patient?'

My management of this patient would depend on the frequency of expectoration, which is increased in this patient. Patients with increased respiratory secretions suffering from atelectasis benefit from simple conservative measures such as sitting the patient upright, and adequate analgesic to encourage deep breathing. I would also involve the physiotherapy team to perform chest physiotherapy, including postural drainage and percussion. I would also encourage the patient to perform deep breathing exercises to help aerate collapsed alveoli. I would monitor the patient closely for signs of improvement. If blood results and chest radiograph results suggested an infection, I would prescribe appropriate antibiotics to combat this. Patient-controlled analgesic in both situations would be beneficial.

Background information

Postoperative atelectasis is an important and common cause for morbidity following surgical intervention. It is partial or complete collapse of the alveoli, resulting in reduced or absent gas exchange in this region of the lungs. A number of factors contribute to atelectasis, and can be considered in terms of increased secretion production secondary to irritation or inflammation and reduced secretion removal:

Increased secretion production:

- Intubation
- Anaesthesia
- Mechanical ventilation
- Underlying lung disease

Reduced secretion removal:

- Inadequate postoperative analgesic
- Upper abdominal incisions
- Reduced mobilisation
- Lying prone
- Smoking history
- Underlying lung disease

With regards to the lung itself, reduced lung compliance, increased and retained airway secretions and reduced spontaneous and depth of breathing all contribute to the occurrence of atelectasis.

Patients with abundant respiratory secretions benefit from interventions that aid in the removal and expulsion of these secretions, such as physiotherapy. Patient suffering from atelectasis who display reduced secretions are more amenable to continuous positive airway pressure, which has been shown to reduce the occurrence of pneumonia, sepsis and hypoxaemia.

Clinical vignettes for further practice

A 32-year-old male undergoes an open appendicectomy procedure. The operation proceeded without complication; postoperatively, however, the patient has complained of ongoing pain. On day 3 following the operation, the nursing staff notice an increase in his temperature and respiratory rate alongside desaturation.

> *Wherever possible incorporate the use of other teams in your management plans. Optimising a patient's diabetic state, mobilising patients with physiotherapists, or asking the advice of a dietician in colorectal surgery patients demonstrates a multi-disciplinary approach to patient care.*

2.33 PR BLEEDING

Clinical case

You are asked to review a 48-year-old female who has presented with bleeding from the back passage. She first noticed this 3 days ago after opening her bowels and on wiping noticed bright red blood on the tissue. She has had several episodes since then. The bleeding is not painful but is now also present in the pan as well as the tissue paper. Clearly embarrassed, the patient also admits to episodes of extreme discomfort around the anus which often feels moist and very itchy.

'How would you proceed with this patient?'

I would first resuscitate the patient and assess her level of health using the ALS protocol A, B, C. Starting with airway, I would speak with the patient and ensure there was a patent airway and no escalation was needed. I would briefly examine the chest for any gross pathologies. For circulation, I would asses the fluids status of the patient by examining the skin turgor, capillary refill, tongue hydration, JVP and signs of peripheral oedema. I would gain intravenous access and examine vital sign monitoring adjuncts. I would examine the patient's cardiovascular system and assess her haemodynamic status. I would react to any abnormal clinical findings and initiate therapy, at which point I would reassess the patient. Once the patient is stable, I would then take a focused history based on the patient's presenting complaint, relevant past medical and drug history as well as social circumstances.

> Do not be fooled by the clinical vignette. It may be a springboard for several avenues of discussion. Remain on your guard when giving answers. Candidates in the past have begun with a general surgery vignette which has ended with a discussion of ENT.

'What are your differentials for this patient?'

My primary diagnosis for this patient would be haemorrhoids supported by the presence of bright red, painless bleeding which usually occurs after the patient opens her bowels. There also appear to be episodes of anal pruritus, which often accompany this condition. I would also consider a rectal prolapse, although this is unlikely based on the demographic of the patient. There may also be an anal fissure, which would more often present as a painful episode of bleeding and is often associated with constipation. Finally, the patient may also have inflammatory bowel disease, although this is usually associated with changes in bowel habits such as diarrhoea.

'What is a haemorrhoid?'

Haemorrhoids are a complication of the anal cushions, which are involved in the control of continence. The cushions are highly vascular tissues that are comprised of arteriovenous anastomosis. These cushions can become dilated, enlarged and congested, eventually protruding as a prolapsed haemorrhoid or 'pile'. The most common cause for this is primarily excessive straining, although any cause of raised intra-abdominal pressure can cause haemorrhoid formation.

'How would you investigate this patient?'

Following resuscitation and a focused history, I would examine the patient's abdomen and perform a digital rectal exam. I would be looking for a palpable anal mass which would represent a prolapsed haemorrhoid. I would then request a FBC to look for signs of anaemia in significantly bleeding patients. An anoscopic examination would be the main stay of the investigation in order to visualise the haemorrhoids. I would take the opportunity to look for skin tags, anal fissures and perianal haematomas. This may form the basis of a colonoscopy investigation to explore other diseases such as inflammatory bowel disease.

'The patient is found to have internal haemorrhoids, what initial treatment options would you offer?'

I would initially begin with conservative treatment centred around dietary and lifestyle changes. This would include an increased fibre diet to reduce the instance of constipation, whilst behavioural changes would include reduced straining and seating time when opening bowels. Since this patient has also presented with pruritus ani, I would also consider short-term corticosteroid injections.

'What other options would you consider if conservative management failed?'

If conservative treatment failed, I would consider more invasive measures ranging from rubber band ligation of the haemorrhoids, injection of sclerosant material, photocoagulation with infra-red radiation or operative management. Rubber band ligation is the most effective treatment, causing necrosis of the haemorrhoid. This is followed by sclerotherapy and photocoagulation, the latter often requires multiple treatment sessions. If these treatments fail, operative management would be stapled haemorrhoidectomy, which is usually reserved for severe haemorrhoid disease.

Background information

Haemorrhoids may be classed as internal or proximal to the dentate line, while external haemorrhoids are distal to the dentate line. They usually present as painless bright red rectal bleeding and are a common surgical presentation. Risk factors include a peak age between 45 and 65 years, constipation and a form of raised intra-abdominal pressure, such as pregnancy or a pelvic mass. Patients most commonly complain of rectal bleeding with perianal discomfort such as pruritus or perianal masses.

Internal haemorrhoid classification:

Grade	Description
1	Haemorrhoid remains bounded with anal canal
2	Protrusion occurs beyond anal canal with spontaneous regression after straining
3	Protrusion occurs beyond anal canal requiring manual reduction
4	Irreducible protrusion beyond the anal canal.

Complications of haemorrhoids include:

- Anaemia secondary to significant or consistent bleeding
- Thrombosis causing perianal pain
- Incarceration of prolapsed haemorrhoids
- Faecal incontinence
- Anal stenosis

Clinical vignettes for further practice

A 32-year-old male complains of severe pain in the anal region for the last 5 days. The pain initially started intermittently but has been increasing in severity, particularly on visiting the bathroom. After going for a run today, the patient suffered exquisite rectal pain. Upon examination, there is a 1 cm by 2 cm blue lesion that is close to the anal canal and extremely painful on palpation.

> Don't forget to re-review the patient. It's really tempting to just reel off a list of interventions like analgesia, NG tubes and that kind of thing. Make sure you tell the interviewer you are going to go back and see the impact of your interventions as well.

2.34 RECTAL PROLAPSE

Clinical case

You are asked to review a 59-year-old female who has suffered a rectal prolapse. The patient has suffered from this before, and has usually been able to reduce the prolapse herself. However, she has been unable to do so on this occasion and saw her GP who has referred her to you. She suffers from constipation and hypertension but is otherwise well. She denies any PR bleeding or other associated symptoms. She is accompanied by her three children who are anxious about her condition.

'What other abnormalities may this patient have?'

Other than a rectal prolapse, I would also wish to investigate prolapsed haemorrhoids which can present in a similar fashion. An important pathology to exclude would be a solitary rectal ulcer though this patient has not complained of any bleeding or passage of mucus.

'What important features would you ask when taking the history and performing your examination?'

This patient appears well versed in recognising when she has suffered a prolapse. I would, however, also check to see if there is any associated bleeding or mucus discharge on defaecation. The patient may have noticed an alteration in her bowel habits, alongside a feeling of abdominal discomfort and incomplete evacuation of bowels. The patient has already mentioned noticing a mass at the rectum in the past and using manual manoeuvres to reduce it. I would like the opportunity to examine the patient in order to review the mass and decide clinically if it was a rectal prolapse or other abnormality such as a haemorrhoid. I would also examine the abdomen and perform a digital rectal examination.

'Why would you perform a digital rectal examination?'

I would be looking for the characteristic concentric rings of the rectum protruding through the anus, as a confirmation of a rectal prolapse. This would need to be reduced. A digital rectal examination would be important to assess for anal sphincter weakness, pelvic floor muscle strength and the presence of any masses.

'Following resuscitation how would you reduce this patients' prolapse?'

I would give the patient adequate analgesic in case of discomfort and before beginning the reduction. I would apply generous amounts of lubricating gel on the prolapse and then gently with firm pressure use my hand to coax and slide the rectum back to its original place. I would not perform this if the prolapse appeared gangrenous, and I would warn the patient that a small amount of discomfort and bleeding may occur. Following reduction, I would ensure all measures to prevent acute constipation had been employed.

'What surgical management could you offer this patient with recurrent prolapse?'

Indications for surgical management include a recurrent rectal prolapse associated with faecal incontinence, constipation and the feeling of a mass at the rectum. There are various different surgical procedures to manage a rectal prolapse, these include rectopexy with or without suture repair, mesh rectopexy and rectopexy with sigmoid resection. A discussion with the patient would be important in order to decide on the most appropriate surgical management.

Background information

A complete rectal prolapse describes the protrusion of the rectum that involves all of its layers – recognisable by the presence of concentric rings. A partial rectal prolapse involves only the mucosa – recognisable by radial folds only. Risk factors for this condition include:

- Female patients aged over 40
- Multiparity
- Vaginal delivery
- Previous pelvic surgery
- Chronic straining behaviour
- Chronic diarrhoea
- Chronic constipation
- Cystic fibrosis
- Dementia
- Stroke
- Pelvic floor dysfunction
- Pelvic floor anatomical defects (e.g. rectocele, cystocele, enterocele)

Medical treatment centres around the reduction of risk factors, including adequate fluid and fibre intake in order to reduce constipation and straining behaviours. Pelvic floor exercises are often recommended although there is limited evidence suggesting their benefit in preventing rectal prolapse at present.

Clinical vignettes for further practice

A 47-year-old female presents following a rectal prolapse that she has been unable to reduce. She suffers from constipation and intermittent diarrhoea. Recently, she has suffered episodes of faecal incontinence.

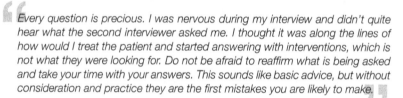

Every question is precious. I was nervous during my interview and didn't quite hear what the second interviewer asked me. I thought it was along the lines of how would I treat the patient and started answering with interventions, which is not what they were looking for. Do not be afraid to reaffirm what is being asked and take your time with your answers. This sounds like basic advice, but without consideration and practice they are the first mistakes you are likely to make.

2.35 SCROTAL SWELLING

Clinical case

You are asked to review a 52-year-old male who has been admitted under medical care. The patient suffers from poorly controlled type 2 diabetes and as a result has chronic kidney disease requiring peritoneal dialysis. He was admitted due to acute on chronic renal failure, with acute abdominal distension and scrotal swelling. He was catheterised with difficulty and is now comfortable. He states the scrotal swelling has been long-standing but has been getting progressively worse since he started dialysis; it is particularly worse towards the end of the day. Upon examination of the scrotal swelling you see the following:

'What are your differentials for this patient?'

My primary diagnosis for this patient would include a hydrocele secondary to peritoneal dialysis. I would also consider an incarcerated inguinoscrotal hernia. Other causes of scrotal swelling may also include varicoceles and testicular tumours.

The clinical station will involve common surgical presentations. Be able to recognise the classical presentations of these pathologies with important variations. The mainstay of questions centres around the correct diagnosis and safe management of these conditions.

'Why might the patient have thickening of the scrotum?'

The patient stated in his history that the scrotal swelling has been long-standing and gradually worsening since the start of peritoneal dialysis. This may have precipitated the formation of a communicating hydrocele. Scrotal oedema will have contributed to the gross enlargement of the scrotum with thickening of the skin layers.

'What are the classic features of a hydrocele?'

The common features of a hydrocele include a scrotal mass, which represents the fluid around the testicle. If this is large, the mass may feel soft on palpation, while a smaller effusion may feel more tense. I would expect variations in the size of the swelling depending on a number of factors including chronicity and cause. Situations causing increased intra-abdominal pressure will cause increased extrusion of fluid toward the scrotal sac, and this would be more typical towards the end of the day compared to the start. Other activities such as coughing and straining would also cause a similar increase in the size of the swelling. Finally, a characteristic sign of a hydrocele would be transillumination, although in long-standing scrotal oedema this may be less obvious.

'What would be the definitive treatment for this patient?'

Although many hydroceles will improve with observation and scrotal support, this patient has a clear cause for which definitive treatment would be operative. The hydrocele can undergo excision or be internally drained with plication of the hydrocele wall layers. In disease associated with filarial infection, complete excision of the tunica vaginalis would be required to prevent recurrence.

'What alternatives could you offer a patient not fit for surgery?'

Alternative treatment options may include aspiration of the hydrocele with sclerotherapy with relative success, although I would warn the patient about post-procedure pain and recurrence. The procedure involves the injection of local anaesthetic followed by insertion of an aspiration needle and drainage of the hydrocele. The sclerosant is injected after this and should be allowed to drain or be reabsorbed.

Background Information

This is an unusual presentation of an otherwise common condition in male children (congenital) and adolescents (acquired), and furthermore an excellent scenario to test a candidate's ability to think about causative factors for a surgical problem. A hydrocele is a collection of serous fluid that accumulates between the surrounding membrane of the testis (tunica vaginalis) or along the spermatic cord. Females may also have this presentation along the canal of Nuck. Risk factors include:

- Male gender
- Premature, low birth weight
- <6 months of age
- Late testicular descension
- Trauma or inflammation within the scrotum
- Testicular cancer
- Connective tissue disorder
- Post varicocelectomy
- Filariasis

In children, surgery is offered if a hydrocele persists beyond the age of 2 years old, otherwise there is an increased risk of incarcerated inguinal hernia. Similarly, in adolescent patients, observation of a hydrocele is offered unless the patient experiences significant discomfort or infection.

Clinical vignettes for further practice

An anxious mother accompanies her 1-year-old male child to A/E after palpating a left-sided scrotal mass. She first noticed the lump while bathing her child and observed it for 3 days; in the morning the mass would disappear, but she then noticed an increase in the size of the left scrotum towards the evening. The mass is not palpable and shines brightly on transillumination.

> *Do not get complacent with your revision of topics. It will always be typical that the few topics you choose to ignore come up in the clinical station. I was not a fan of urology and thought I had escaped when I read the clinical vignette. During the station, however, the discussions in between the clinical vignette involved adult and paediatric presentations in urology which I struggled with.*

2.36 SWOLLEN PENIS

Clinical case

You are asked to review a 3-year-old male referred by the paediatric team. The child is accompanied by his mother who describes bathing her child the night before. She had noticed that retracting the foreskin was always moderately difficult, but had mostly ignored the problem. She was able to retract the foreskin yesterday, with a degree of force, and had left the foreskin retracted. The child has been in pain since, and the foreskin appears oedematous and does not return to its original position.

'How would you proceed with this patient?'

I would begin by resuscitating the patient and assess his level of health using the ALS protocol A, B, C. Once stabilised, I would alert my senior that I was examining a child of this given age and proceed to clarify the history of the patient with his mother. I would undertake an examination in a calm relaxed environment, preferably with a chaperone alongside the patient's mother.

The interviewers are not looking for ready-made surgical registrars. Your knowledge base provides you with an opportunity to demonstrate excellence but communication skills, patient safety, working with colleagues, and so on, is far more important and you should practise demonstrating this in your answers.

'What specific features in the history and examination would you elicit?'

This patient may be suffering from a paraphimosis for which I would first consider risk factors such as tight foreskin, poor hygiene, previous infections and trauma to the penis. I would then enquire about penile pain, problems when retracting the foreskin and urinating. Upon examination, I would look for a band of retracted foreskin below the glans of the penis, and a swollen penile glans which often has an accompanying collar of oedematous foreskin. Finally, I would examine for erythema, exquisite pain and any red flag signs such as gangrene, necrosis and a non-pliable penis glans.

'How would you investigate this patient?'

The diagnosis in this patient is largely clinical, I would therefore avoid any invasive and unnecessary investigations, especially in a child. A urine dipstick would be helpful to ensure no concomitant urinary tract infection was present. I would only consider taking bloods if there were any worrying features, such as sepsis.

'How would you treat this patient?'

Following stabilisation, I would first try to reassure and calm the patient with distraction techniques and keeping the mother close by. Assuming there were no red flag signs, I would place topical analgesic agents around the penis and consider using ice-packs, with the penis protected, to reduce the swelling. I would proceed with compression of the swollen area using gloved hand manipulation. If this is too painful, or initially fails, I would consider applying an osmotic agent such as concentrated dextrose or sugar in large amounts over the swollen area to create an osmotic effect. I would re-attempt manipulation following this, and if the area of swelling has improved significantly, I would manually reduce the glans penis whilst pulling the foreskin back over it.

'If your attempts fail what other interventions would you consider?'

If conservative management fails, I would discuss the patient and my progress with a senior who may consider employing the puncture maneouvre – whereby the foreskin is punctured in multiple areas and then compressed – to allow for the oedema to be expelled and a reduction of the paraphimosis. Should this also fail, surgical reduction in the theatre can be considered, although this would need senior discussion involving the parent, who would understandably need reassurance. In the theatre manual compression can be attempted again, although at this stage, performing a dorsal slit and allowing oedema to be exuded is more common. Once the swelling has disappeared, the edges can be closed and an elective circumcision planned with a paediatric urologist.

Background information

A paraphimosis can affect any male age group, but is often most challenging when occurring in young children. It most often results when engorgement of a retracted foreskin causes swelling and tightening around the glans. Circumcision is the most successful preventative measure against the occurrence of a paraphimosis. In older patients who have indwelling catheters, patients and carers should be advised that a retracted foreskin should be returned to its natural position without excessive force. Other risk factors include indwelling catheterisation, poor hygiene, phimosis, recurrent infections of the area, piercings, diabetes and trauma. Patients presenting with ischaemia or necrosis require emergency surgery with a urology consultant who will try to reduce the offending tissue. Gangrenous or necrosed skin will undergo debridement.

Clinical vignettes for further practice

A 71-year-old male is referred from a nursing home after carers noticed the patient being agitated following a catheter change. The patient suffers from diabetes, vascular dementia and urinary incontinence. He has had several episodes of retention and has a long-term catheter. Upon examination, the foreskin is grossly swollen and retracted, and painful on palpation.

> Having done A/E, I had seen a lot of acute surgical presentations and during my interview the vignette was about general surgery but after this the other interviewer covered ENT, orthopaedics and vascular surgery. It can be daunting to cover material in other specialties but common presentations seen as an SHO or registrar are all you should focus on.

2.37 TESTICULAR SWELLING

Clinical case

As the CT1 in surgery on call, you are asked to see a 22-year-old male urged to attend A/E by his girlfriend. He states that over a 2-month period he has noticed an increasingly heavy and dragging feeling around the scrotum. He is an avid swimmer and apart from asthma suffers no other medical problems. He does not smoke or drink alcohol in excess and denies any fever, urinary symptoms or significant weight loss. Upon examination there is a painless, hard, irregularly shaped mass on the right testicle.

'What is your primary diagnosis in this patient?'

My primary concern would be this patient may have a testicular malignancy given the characteristic history presentation and patient demographics, which support clinical examination findings. I would wish to ensure the patient was not suffering from a testicular torsion, epididymo-orchitis or epididymal cyst.

'What types of testicular cancer do you know?'

Testicular tumours may be primary or secondary. Primary cancers may be further split into germ cell cancers or non-germ cell. The germ-cell tumours represent the majority of primary testicular cancers and include seminoma and teratoma. Non-germ cell tumours include Leydig cell tumours. Secondary cancers include metastases such as lymphomas.

'What extra-testicular features would you ask about?'

I would ask the patient if they had noticed any features of bone pain, typically in the lower back and spine, which may represent skeletal metastases. I would also ask if the patient has noticed other lumps or lesions, specifically lymph nodes in the groin and supra-clavicular region. I would also examine for gynaecomastia which may arise from byproducts of the testicular malignancy.

'What specific investigations would you consider for this patient?'

Alongside other investigations, I would request a serum beta-hCG, which is increased in all cases of choriocarcinoma and suggestive of seminoma. Alpha-fetoprotein is elevated in combined tumours and directs away from choriocarinoma and seminomas. Finally, with regards to serum tests, the lactate dehydrogenase is increased in approximately 50% of all testicular malignancies. My mainstay of investigation would be an ultrasound scan which is highly sensitive.

'How would you proceed if the patient's tumour markers were elevated, but the US scan was normal?'

In this situation, I would consider a CT scan of the abdomen and pelvis, which may detect abnormal masses missed on US scan, as well as identify enlarged lymph nodes. Alongside this, a CXR would be helpful to identify mediastinal and lung metastases. If these were positive a CT scan of the chest could be performed.

'What would be the safest way to perform histology investigations on the testicular mass?'

The safest method would be to perform a radical inguinal orchidectomy and send the tissue for histology. A biopsy – although more convenient – would not be safe as it risks spreading the malignant cells or 'seeding'.

Background information

Testicular tumours most commonly present as hard painless masses typically on a single testicle and are noticed incidentally. Optimal investigations include elevated serum tumour markers, alongside positive US scan results. Seminomas are the most common germ cell malignancies and their treatment involves radiation therapy post-orchidectomy, which can be supplemented with systemic chemotherapy in more advanced disease. Non-seminomas benefit from retroperitoneal lymph node dissection post-orchidectomy, which again can be supplemented with combination chemotherapy in more advanced disease.

Clinical vignettes for further practice

A 30-year-old male presents with non-specific pains in the lower back alongside a 1-month history of non-productive cough. He has noticed a dragging sensation in the scrotal area, but has not found any suspicious masses on examination.

> *Bring multidisciplinary teams into your answer when this makes sense and fits in with the question being asked. It can seem silly at first but sounds really impressive. Instead of just requesting an ultrasound, I said I would also go to the radiologist and see the scans and get his/her advice about the results. This shows your ability to go the extra step and easily sets you ahead of other people at interview.*

2.38 URINARY RETENTION

Clinical case

You are asked to see a 66-year-old male who has had increasing difficulty in passing urine. He admits to frequency, nocturia and dysuria despite multiple treatments with antibiotics. This morning on waking, he was unable to pass urine and has continued to be in retention for the last 8 hours. He is otherwise fit and well. Upon examination, there is suprapubic pain and a palpable bladder. His observations are within normal range, except for heart rate which is 100 bpm.

'What other details would you elicit from the examination?'

In addition to the vignette, I would examine for renal angle tenderness, which in an apyrexial patient would suggest an obstruction, signs of neurological disease such as spinal cord injury or signs suggestive of multiple sclerosis. I would perform a PR examination to document anal tone response. I would also wish to document the characteristics of the prostate gland specifically to palpate for an enlargement, which suggests benign prostatic hypertrophy, or a dysmorphic and craggy prostate suggestive of malignancy. I would also inspect the genitalia to look for meatal narrowing.

'What are the causes of urinary obstruction?'

Differential	Explanation
BPH	Prostatic hypertrophy can cause acute uni- and bilateral obstruction
Iatrogenic	Alpha receptor antagonists, anticholinergics
Ureteric calculi	Stones <5 mm are more likely to pass without consequence
Neurological	Parkinson's, spinal cord injury, multiple sclerosis
Malignancy	Prostate, bladder, cervix and colon
Meatal stenosis	Evident on clinical examination or attempted catheterisation

'What investigation would you perform for this patient?'

I would begin with a urine analysis using a urine dipstick to look for positive leukocytes, nitrites and haematuria. Obstruction complicated by infection would need prompt intervention. For bloods, I would request an FBC to look for anaemia, raised WCC and neutrophils suggesting an infection. I would look at urea and electrolytes to examine for raised urea and creatinine, suggesting renal failure or hydronephrosis. A PSA test may also be helpful in this patient who is likely suffering from BPH, but also perhaps a more sinister pathology. For more invasive tests, I would consider a renal ultrasound to support renal compromise secondary to an obstructive cause. A CT KUB is ideal for patients with a history suggestive of a renal stone.

'How would you manage this patient?'

I would begin by formally resuscitating the patient myself, and assessing his level of health using the ALS protocol A, B, C. Following a focused history and examination, I would make the patient comfortable with appropriate analgesic and ensuring the patient had no allergies. I would then attempt to insert a urinary catheter, sized appropriately for the patient, under aseptic conditions with prophylactic antibiotic cover if there are signs of urinary infection and if the renal function permits it. If successful, I would examine the urinary content, volume and character. In the event the catheterisation is unsuccessful, a differently sized catheter can be used with the use of an introducer – if I felt safe and competent to do so. If I felt unsafe or remained unsuccessful, I would consider a suprapubic catheter insertion under supervision. At all times, I would ensure the patient was well supported and not under undue discomfort.

If a suprapubic catheter is also unsuccessful, preparations could be made for a catheter insertion under cystoscopy guidance.

'An US scan shows an obstructed stone secondary to a calculus with signs of sepsis. How would you now proceed?'

I would again ensure that the patient had adequate analgesic and was being hydrated through intravenous infusion. I would progress with pain relief in a step-wise manner, along the WHO recommended pain ladder, though initially with more robust analgesic such as ketorolac alongside alpha blockage with tamsulosin. Since there are also signs of sepsis, I would initiate appropriate antibiotics to begin treating this with a combined regimen – based on blood and urinary results – such as ciprofloxacin and gentamicin. I would consult the hospital regulated policy and seniors as appropriate. Finally, I would discuss the results with the patient, and alongside a senior begin preparations for the insertion of a ureteric stent or nephrostomy to drain the kidney.

Background information

Urinary retention may result depending on the level of obstruction within the urinary tract. The most common conditions causing an obstruction include urolithiasis and benign prostatic hypertrophy. Alongside pain relief and fluid resuscitation of the patient, an obstruction can lead to hydronephrosis eventually causing significant renal injury. Relief of the back pressure is imperative to prevent permanent damage from occurring, and this may be carried out through catheterisation, stent insertion or a nephrostomy.

Important differentials to consider include:

- Hydronephrosis secondary to pregnancy
- Abdominal aortic aneurysm
- Ovarian pathology
- Bowel obstruction

In patients with calculi <10 mm, one can resuscitate with analgesic and fluid therapy in the hope that the stone passes, thereby relieving symptoms as well as the obstruction. This can be aided with the addition of tamsulosin or alfuzosin, which may improve stone passage in up to 20% of patients. If these measures fail, intervention is then required in order to relieve the obstruction. This may be in a number of forms such as lithotripsy or percutaneous nephrolithotomy. In larger stones >10 mm, intervention is more readily offered due to the unlikely chance of stone passage.

In obstruction secondary to benign prostatic hypertrophy first line management is catheterisation. For urethral strictures, a smaller silicone catheter or suprapubic catheter can be considered. BPH itself can be overcome using a curved tip or 'Coude' catheter. If this fails, a more experienced practitioner must then usually consider catheterisation using an introducer, suprapubic catheterisation or cystoscopy. This can be supplemented with prophylactic antibiotics, alpha blockade and the use of 5-alpha reductase inhibitors such as finasteride.

Clinical vignettes for further practice

A 45-year-old male presents to A/E with acute urinary retention. He has been complaining of a colicky loin to groin pain for the last 6 hours. He feels nauseated and has vomited once whilst in the department. A urine dipstick is positive for haematuria, leukocytes and nitrites.

> *I kept forgetting where I left off my vignette patient while answering other questions. I said I would begin taking bloods and then answered a question about trauma. When I came back to the vignette I repeated myself but was steered back to where I left off. They were both fair to me in the interview.*

2.39 VOMITING CHILD

Clinical case

You are referred a 4-week-old male infant who has been brought to A/E by his parents concerned about his increasing vomiting behaviour following feeding. They were initially breast feeding and then switched to formula feeding in an attempt to alleviate the problem. They deny any bile in the vomitus. They have become particularly anxious as the vomiting now occurs regularly after feeding and is often forceful. The infant was delivered naturally at term with no issues at the time of birth.

'What are your differentials for this patient?'

My primary diagnosis would be pyloric stenosis, as evidenced by the consistent vomiting after feeds alongside the young demographics of the patient. Other possibilities include pyloric or duodenal atresia, overfeeding and gastro-oesophageal reflux disease.

Maintain a low threshold for escalation and treatment in children. They have an excellent capacity for compensation, sick children may often appear relatively normal before physiological collapse. You should have a basic knowledge of fluid calculations. We include them here because of their importance in looking after paediatric patients properly.

'What would you be most concerned about this child?'

Pyloric stenosis is characterised by persistent vomiting after feeds, which is often described as projectile. This would lead to a worrying loss of fluid and electrolytes, eventually causing hypovolaemia and a hypochloraemic, hypokalaemic metabolic alkalosis.

'What diagnostic features in the history and examination would you elicit?'

The occurrence of non-bilious vomiting after feeds is a cardinal presentation, patients tend to be young presenting within 6 weeks of birth in term children. The parents may state multiple formula changes and also increasing irritability of the child. There may be visible peristaltic waves representing gastric contractions. Upon palpation, an olive-shaped mass may also be present. I would be particularly concerned by features such as decreasing wet nappies, constipation, poor weight gain and failing to meet growth targets. These features would suggest severe hypovolaemia. Upon examination, I would review basic observations to look for a tachycardia, low blood pressure, and increased respiration rate.

'What clinical signs would you assess to estimate level of dehydration?'

I would assess objective signs such as the pulse, systolic blood pressure, respiration rate and urine output. Upon examination, I would assess the buccal mucosa, anterior fontanelle and various other mucous membranes including the eyes, skin turgor and skin appearance. Objective signs that would suggest severe dehydration would include a weak pulse, low blood pressure, low urine output and tachypnoea. Worrying features of the mucous membranes would include dry buccal mucosa, sunken eyes and fontanelles, lethargic reactions and mottling of the skin.

'How would you treat this patient?'

Depending on the level of dehydration this patient may require emergency treatment. I would alert the A/E team for assistance and contact a senior in surgery and, ideally, a member of the paediatric team. I would move the patient to a paediatric resuscitation bay and assess his level of health using the ALS protocol A, B, C. I would speak with the patient's parents and ensure there was a patent airway, also examine the chest for gross pathologies. For circulation, I would assess the patient's level of fluid loss as mild, moderate or severe. I would proceed with intravenous access which, if difficult or prolonged, may necessitate intraosseous access; following this, I would send away routine bloods along with a group and save sample, plasma glucose and electrolytes. I would then initiate fluid resuscitation of the patient and assess the need for a nasogastric tube to reduce further instances of vomiting.

'In severe dehydration what would be your approach to fluid resuscitation?'

I would first rectify the patient's losses and prescribe a 20 mL/kg fluid bolus of normal saline or Hartmann's solution infused over 5–10 mins. I would repeat this action with reassessment up to three times if there was no improvement and no signs of fluid overload. Once the patient had begun to recover, I would then estimate the patient's fluid deficit (10 × weight in kg × % dehydration) and prescribe an appropriate volume of normal saline over 24 hours. I would monitor the patient's response closely and ensure all decisions were approved by a senior first.

'Would you prescribe the patient any more fluids in addition to their fluid loss?'

Yes, the patient would require maintenance fluid infusion alongside their fluid loss replacement. I would calculate this by prescribing 100 mL/kg/24 hours for the patient's first 10 kg, 50 mL/kg/24 hours for the next 10 kg and finally 20 mL/kg/24 hours for every kilogram exceeding 20 kg. I would again monitor the patient's response closely and ensure all decisions were approved by a senior first.

'What is the definitive management of this patient after stabilisation?'

Following adequate resuscitation, the patient would require a pyloromyotomy which corrects the gastric outlet obstruction caused by pyloric hypertrophy; this may be offered as an open or laparoscopic procedure.

Background information

Pyloric stenosis resulting in persistent vomiting is considered a surgical emergency due to the rapid descent into hypovolaemic shock. Patients typically present within 6 weeks of birth and most often have a history of multiple feeding modality changes and post-feeding vomiting. The exact causes of pyloric hypertrophy remain unclear, with multiple causative factors. Risk factors include first born male patients, a family history of pyloric stenosis and some suggestion that macrolide exposure can predispose to pyloric stenosis. Clinical examination and US scan form the mainstay of investigation with high sensitivity.

Indications for intravenous fluid therapy include:

- Inability of the child to accept oral rehydration (e.g. vomiting, ileus, anatomical anomalies or mental state compromise)
- Oral rehydration failing to provide adequate rehydration (e.g. persistent vomiting)
- Severe electrolyte derangement

The table that follows is a guide for estimating the percentage of clinical dehydration.

Finding	Mild (3%–5%)	Moderate (6%–9%)	Severe (≥10%)
Pulse	Normal	Tachycardia	Tachycardia, weak or absent
Blood pressure	Normal	Normal to low	Low
Respirations	Normal	Tachypnoea	Tachypnoeic or reduced
Buccal mucosa	Slightly dry	Dry	Parched
Anterior fontanelle	Normal	Sunken	Severely sunken
Eyes	Normal	Sunken	Severely sunken

Skin turgor	Normal	Reduced	Mottled
Urine output	Normal	Reduced	Anuric
Systemic signs	Normal	Irritable	Lethargic

Clinical vignettes for further practice

A 3-week-old male infant is brought in semi-conscious by his father into the A/E reception. You attend to the patient along with the junior doctors in A/E. The father states the child has been vomiting persistently after feeds, and in the last 2 days has had dry nappies and reduced bowel movements. Upon examination the child is extremely drowsy with markedly sunken eyes and mottled skin.

It's tempting to suggest you have seen every pathology the interviewers ask you about. It helps to draw from the experience but be honest. If you haven't seen a particular pathology be honest and answer based on theory that you do know. I had seen pyloric stenosis patients during my paediatric surgery rotation, but had never examined them properly before. The interviewer asked me if I had examined such patients in depth and I said that I had. They then proceeded to ask about my examination findings and it was obvious I knew textbook answers rather than from live experience. Be honest and truthful at all times.

3. INTRODUCTION TO THE MANAGEMENT STATION

The management interview station is often overlooked by candidates at their peril. You must remember that each of the three stations is equally important and you should aim to excel in all sections of the interview. This station challenges your ability to deal with professional and non-clinical issues that arise at work. As a core surgical trainee, you will have more responsibility not only from seniors but towards more junior members of your team. As a result, you should be aware of the procedures and boundaries that govern professional conduct. The format of this station is variable and you may be given a vignette within the station around which various discussions can be formulated, or you may be asked more direct questions. As before, your articulation of answers is paramount and you will be assessed on your communication ability as well as the content of your answers. Many candidates will not be knowledgeable about this area of clinical practice. There is important factual information that you should be aware of which we have included in this guide, whilst in other sections you will be challenged in ethically ambiguous situations.

For broad topic based discussions use the SALE answer structure (Surgical, Academic, Leadership and Extracurricular). For more challenging scenarios you will find the SCAM (Scenario, Context, Appraisal and Management) and SCAPES (Scenario description, Context of events, Appraisal of dangers, Patient safety, Escalation and Senior support) structures more helpful.

> The management station is a difficult station to approach and it is essential that you do some reading around various topics. There will be information in Good Medical Practice that helps you decide what the most appropriate course of action is. As an example, explaining what an audit cycle is, is relatively easy but explaining why clinical audits are important requires knowledge and understanding of clinical governance first.

Once again, where appropriate, you can draw from your past experiences in situations that you have been in to aid your answer. Reviewing your log of reflections is an invaluable resource, and we encourage you to review these as they are representative of some of the scenarios upon which you will be interviewed. At all times utilise the information in this section to demonstrate you understand the principles behind safe and professional clinical conduct.

3.1 BAD COMMUNICATION

'Can you describe a difficult experience when communicating with a patient?'

During a busy on-call week in surgery our team was placed in a difficult situation. A patient under treatment for colorectal carcinoma had begun to suffer from non-specific respiratory symptoms. A specialised scan was organised and we, along with the patient, were awaiting the report. The patient was understandably impatient about his results and would continually ask for the report. There was an unfortunate communication error between a senior member of the team and the patient who was led to believe they would receive the results on a given day. The patient's family therefore made a long journey to the hospital to support the patient who was understandably annoyed along with his family that no results were forthcoming. The senior members of the team were all busy in the theatre for the whole day, and therefore, I was asked to speak to the patient and his family.

'How did this affect you?'

I was placed in a difficult position since I had not directly been involved in the initial communication with the patient. I also did not have any further news regarding the outcome of the report, or when it may become available. Since the senior members of the team were busy with emergency cases in the theatre, it would not be fair to keep the patient and his family waiting without some form of address.

'How did you resolve this situation?'

I spoke to the other members of the team and ensured that I could be excused to speak to the family. I then spoke to the family to confirm this meeting. I completed my pending jobs before this time and then handed over the bleep to another team member so that we wouldn't be disturbed. I also spoke to the nursing staff and requested we not be disturbed for a period of time. The patient was in a quiet and spacious side room and was happy to stay here with the relatives for the discussion. On entering, I introduced myself again to the patient explaining who I was and my role with the surgical team. I also identified everyone else in the room, their relation to the patient and introduced myself to them also. I began by apologising to everyone about the inconvenience caused, as well as for the anxiety they must have all been through. I explained the miscommunication that had occurred from our team and again apologised for the inaccurate information. I spent time listening to the patient and his family express their grievance, however, they were very grateful that a team member had organised an uninterrupted period to speak to them personally. I explained the current situation and the action that I would take after speaking with them. On ending the consultation, I thanked everyone again for their time and then documented the conversation in the patient's notes. I included details of everyone in the room, the details of the conversation and the agreed action plan. I also relayed this information to the senior members of the team who also arranged a time to speak with the patient and their family. Finally, I reflected on this episode and created an anonymised entry in my portfolio. I listed the scenario and the learning points that I had gained from the situation.

Background information

There will be many episodes whereby poor communication has resulted in a conflict between a patient or even a colleague. You may be asked to give an example of this and how you resolved the situation. It is therefore very helpful to review your reflective practice examples and keep the examples to recall from. Demonstrate your level of organisation and consideration by communication with your team and allied health care professionals. Meticulous documentation and using the situation to further your professional development is a good example of maturity that the interviewers will look for.

3.2 CLINICAL GOVERNANCE

'What is clinical governance?'

Clinical governance is a system based upon seven pillars which aim to improve the standard of clinical practice. This was first mentioned in an NHS white paper in 2000, and put in place as a consequence to the Bristol Heart and Harold Shipman enquiries. It ensures that clinical standards are maintained with continuous improvement.

'What are the seven pillars of clinical governance?'

'CARPETS'

- **C**linical effectiveness and research
- **A**udit
- **R**isk management
- **P**atient and public involvement/openness
- **E**ducation and training
- **T**echnology
- **S**taff management

'What is clinical effectiveness?'

Clinical effectiveness describes the extent to which a particular treatment, service or intervention achieved its desired effect. The National Institute of Clinical Excellence (NICE) is one example which assesses the effectiveness of proposed medical treatments and validates those that are considered clinically effective and financially viable. The Royal College of Surgeons has a clinical effectiveness unit which performs relevant clinical audits and provides evidence regarding cost effectiveness. Interventions and services are based on strong evidence from reviews and statistical findings. These include 'numbers needed to treat' which demonstrate improved clinical practice or service delivery and are considered to be clinically effective. This can be difficult when assessing the qualitative features of a given treatment, such as care that is sensitive and responsive to an individual patient's requirements. Clinical effectiveness in part also encompasses the use of information technology to make clinical practice more efficient.

'What is risk management?'

This is the estimation of providing healthcare and the risks this can have to the patient, the provider and the organisation. Any treatment, intervention or service given to a patient has inherent risks associated with it. In order to minimise these risks, systems are in place to respond to patients' complaints, protect their statutory rights and identify potentially hazardous actions. This includes among many others, the Patient Advice and Liason team (PALS), the Data Protection Act and Control of Substances Hazardous to Heath (COSHH). Risks to providers include, among others, transmitted infections and injuries sustained whilst working (e.g., needle stick injuries). These again can be minimised by ensuring up-to-date vaccinations, safe working environments and protocols for practitioner protection against injuries sustained in the work place. Finally, risk management for organisations entails ensuring the service provision adheres to the highest quality standard and patient safety is maintained at all times. All members of the organisation must agree to comply with these policies.

'What does research and development entail?'

The translation of quality research and its incorporation into mainstream clinical practice is a crucial and challenging obstacle. Clinical care must respond to emerging evidence from clinical research in order to provide the very best healthcare for patients. This can be implemented through thorough critical appraisal of the literature, and the development of guidelines and protocols.

'Why is public and patient involvement important?'

The Bristol Inquiry and Shipman Inquiry demonstrated the danger of operating behind closed doors. As part or in relation to clinical governance and quality assurance aspects of healthcare which can be justified as being in the public interest are eligible for public review whilst maintaining confidentiality of all parties.

'Why is education and training important?'

Continuing professional development is an essential aspect of maintaining a licence to practice. The rapid progression of clinical knowledge often means that medical training can become outdated soon after acquisition. It is a professional duty of all practitioners to remain up to date. Parts of this continuing educational development is the responsibility of the trust for which central funding is available, whilst other specialties require additional or updated training as a prerequisite before entry. This also forms an important basis for staff management.

3.3 CLINICAL INCIDENT REPORTING

'You review the drug card of a sick patient you are concerned about. They are receiving intravenous antibiotics for sepsis, however you notice that the method of administration has been changed from intravenous to oral. You are informed one of the locum nursing staff made this change without any discussion with any team member. How would you proceed?'

This is a potentially serious clinical incident that has put the patient at risk, since they are not receiving the advised treatment. I would clarify the events and ensure I was reading the correct patient's drug chart and that I had understood the changes that had been made to the prescription. I would read the patient's notes to see if there was any documentation from any member of the team looking after the patient that may explain the circumstances. I would also seek to speak to the nursing staff, especially the nurse who had allegedly changed the drug prescription, and confirm this was how the prescription had been changed. Once I had clarified the situation, I would then ensure the patient was safe and attend to him/her first. I would make any safe changes to rectify their treatment plan and review their progress. Finally, I would document this incident in the notes and seek to escalate the incident by informing a senior member of the team and on-call line at the earliest opportunity.

'Your consultant investigates this matter and asks you to complete a clinical incident report. What would this involve?'

Hospitals may have different versions of clinical incident reporting though in each the general principle is the same. I would use a paper incident reporting form or an online version such as Datixweb, depending on what was available to record the details of the incident and those involved. This would include the person affected by the incident, a comprehensive and accurate account of the incident and any supporting witnesses or accounts. I would ensure the date and time were documented and this report was completed within the time frame of the shift and, ideally, as close as possible to the event itself.

'How are clinical incident reports generally processed?'

Again, this may vary but the general principle is similar across trusts. Several copies of the incident report would be made and distributed to appropriate team members and departments. This would include the risk management department (green page), the line manager responsible (yellow page), the national patient safety agency (NPSA) and a separate copy to be kept in a confidential file (white page). The datix system would be similarly reviewed by a risk and line manager before being uploaded to the National Reporting and Learning System (NRLS) – a database operated by the national patient safety agency NPSA. The NPSA supports the NHS to learn from patient safety incidents and consider solutions to prevent similar incidents occurring in the future.

Background information

There is a clear dichotomy of clinical incident reporting between nurses and doctors. Nursing staff are usually very meticulous in recording clinical incidents and well versed in this procedure, whilst doctors are historically very poor.

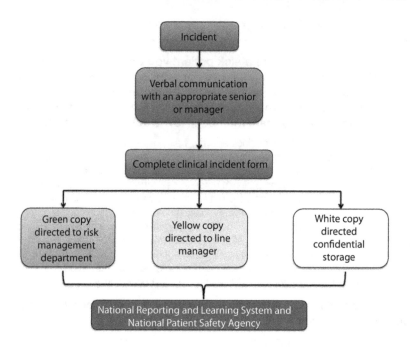

3.4 CONSENT

'Before the morning operating list your consultant asks you to gain consent from a patient who is first on the list for a simple procedure that you have performed before and are aware of the risks and complications. The patient arrives late and is visibly upset having learned their relative has become sick. How would you proceed?'

This is an unfortunate situation in which the patient has arrived in a perturbed frame of mind. The prospect of surgical intervention can be daunting for most patients and the Department of Health, Good Medical Practice and the GMC state that a patient should undertake consent in advance of their procedure in a calm and collected frame of mind. This allows them time to consider the benefits, risks and complications of the procedure and reflect on their decisions. In this situation, therefore, I would not be comfortable obtaining consent as the patient is in a vulnerable state and the procedure is ready to occur imminently. I would attend to the patient first and move them to a quiet private room. I would inform the nursing staff of the situation and then speak to my consultant at the earliest opportunity. I would document the circumstances in the patient's notes and ensure that no preoperative medication was started.

'The theatre staff re-organise the operating list and a different patient is operated on. You are contacted by the theatre staff to consent the next patient on the list in order to save time, as the senior staff are still busy in theatre. The next procedure is more complex and you have limited knowledge regarding the benefits and risks. How would you proceed?'

Once again, this is a difficult situation as the theatre staff and consultant may now be under pressure to advance through the list more efficiently due to the earlier delay. It is not always feasible for the doctor performing the intervention to always gain consent from the patient as advised by the GMC. However, since I have limited knowledge regarding the procedure itself, its indications, benefits and risks, I would once again not be in a comfortable or in a viable position to gain consent from the patient. The patient may wish to know more about their procedure, especially in more complex operations, and I would not be able to give them any advice or knowledge in this regard. I would once again inform the nursing staff in charge of the patient in the preoperative period that I would be speaking to the consultant first. I would then contact the theatre staff and ask if a message could be relayed to the operating team when they are not busy that I would like to speak to the consultant regarding consenting the patient. I would then wait patiently outside the operating theatre, so as not to disturb the on-going procedure.

'How would you assess the capacity of a patient before gaining consent?'

If I had concerns regarding the capacity of a patient I would make an assessment based upon the principles outlined in the Mental Capacity Act 2005. I would ensure the patient and I were in a private setting to begin with. I would then inform the patient's about the procedure including the indications, benefits and risks. I would then assess the patient's ability to understand this information, including the potential consequences of the procedure itself along with a decision not to undertake the treatment. I would appraise the patient's ability to retain the information I had given and then use it to make a balanced and informed decision. Finally, I would complete my assessment based on the patient's ability to communicate their decision back to me. If I had any doubts or concerns regarding a patient's capacity, I would document this carefully in the notes and inform the consultant in charge. It is likely that the involvement of the patient's family, senior staff and other multidisciplinary teams may be required.

'What is Gillick competence?'

Gillick competence describes a judgment made in the high court, in 1983, that provided guidance for children who may demonstrate enough capacity to provide valid consent to treatment. In the United Kingdom, the age distinction between an adult who has full autonomy for their decisions is 18, assuming that they do not lack capacity. For children who are 16 or 17, valid consent may also be obtained independent from the supervision of their parents, strictly assessed on their competence and capacity to fully understand the decisions they are asked to make. A 'Gillick competent' child therefore refers specifically to a patient under the age of 16 legally consenting to medical examination and treatment without parental consent. This is dependent on them being able to display sufficient maturity and competence to fully understand their investigation or treatment. Until a patient reaches the age of 18, regardless of Gillick competence, they may not refuse life-saving treatment performed in their best interest.

'What is the difference between Fraser and Gillick competence?'

Lord Fraser's guidance has a narrower remit to consent, and addresses the specific issue of contraception to ensure that a patient seeking contraception appreciates advice relating to this; but it also highlights the involvement of parents and the risks of unprotected sex.

'Can a Gillick competent patient refuse treatment?'

Current UK Law allows a carer, with parental responsibility, to override a Gillick competent decision of refusal to consent. Similarly, if a Gillick competent child provides consent, this cannot be overruled and refused by a carer with parental responsibility.

Background information

Gaining consent is a mandatory legal obligation that every patient has a right to, and which every practitioner must gain prior to any form of treatment or intervention. The GMC has provided clear guidance in their 2008 publication 'Consent: patients and doctors making decisions together'. Patients may refuse treatment if they have proved capacity, regardless of whether the decision is against their best interest. The GMC advises the following information be given to the patient when gaining consent:

1. Their diagnosis and prognosis including uncertainties and alternative treatments.
2. Options for further investigations.
3. The purpose of any investigations or treatment and what they will involve.
4. The potential benefits, risks and complications, and the likelihood of success, for each option.
5. Whether a proposed investigation or treatment is part of a research programme or is an innovative treatment designed specifically for their benefit.
6. The people who will be mainly responsible for and involved in their care, what their roles are, and to what extent students may be involved.
7. Their right to refuse to take part in teaching or research.
8. Their right to seek a second opinion.
9. Any bills they will have to pay.
10. Any conflicts of interest that you, or your organisation, may have.

Consent issues around children are very common and it is essential that this is well understood. Within the United Kingdom, British courts refer to an individual who is over 18 years of age as adults, 16–17 year olds as young persons, and children as being those under the age of 16. In Scotland only, a child becomes adult once they reach the age of 16, however, guidance does exist to protect children and young people up to the age of 18. Consent law describes a person's journey to gaining full autonomy as passing through three key development stages:

1. The first stage is a child who relies on a carer with parental responsibility to act in their best interests when consenting for treatment or investigation. Any child under the age of 13 may not give legal consent.

2. A child under the age of 16 who displays sufficient maturity may be considered Gillick competent, and in specific situations of contraception they may display Fraser competence.

3. A young person of 16 or 17 may consent to treatment as if they were already of adult age and maturity, after age 16/17 capacity is presumed unless evidence can be shown otherwise. Consent is therefore sought from a patient aged 16 or 17, rather than from a parent or carer.

The medical team must consider acting in a patient's best interest if they are aged over 18, consent cannot be given by those with parental responsibility.

3.5 DISPUTE WITH COLLEAGUE

'A new doctor temporarily replaces a sick member of the surgical team. You notice that your colleagues act in a belittling manner and unfairly distribute jobs unfavourably towards the new member of the team. The new doctor seems despondent and much less enthusiastic than when he/ she first started. How would you deal with this?'

This appears to be an unacceptable situation of bullying. Working as a coherent team with mutual respect between team members is an essential and mandatory aspect of working with colleagues. I would begin by clarifying and confirming the behaviour of my colleagues toward the new doctor. I would objectively review their behaviour and place into context their decisions, communication and behaviour and appraise the evidence that suggests they are acting in an unfair manner. I would also analyse my own behaviour and actions to ensure I was not also contributing to the problem. I would also speak to the new doctor in a private setting and ask them how they felt they were settling into their new post, and whether they felt they were treated as a respected and equal member of the team. Following these actions, I would then highlight those situations that appeared to be unfair to my colleagues (e.g., unreasonable job distribution) and see if they were aware of their actions. I would want to identify episodes where my colleagues appeared to belittle the new doctor and raise them with the team members in a calm, non-aggressive manner to see if they were aware of their actions. It may be possible to resolve this situation locally, whereby my colleagues may not have been aware of how they were treating the new doctor, and take active steps to ensure this behaviour stopped. I would however maintain an extremely low threshold for raising this to a senior member of the team, as I may not be in the best position to deal with colleagues – at my level – who are treating another team member unfairly. I would therefore document my conversations with the new doctor and my colleagues, and formally approach my registrar and/or consultant with my concerns. I would show them objective evidence to support my claims, as this is a serious matter which is likely to affect the doctor's personal performance, and may have an impact on patient care. During my conversation with the new doctor, I would make them aware that this is the action I would consider, but would respect their privacy and confidentiality in personal matters (e.g., their feelings and emotions). I would also reflect on this matter in my e-portfolio, as it will raise several learning points that will further my professional development.

Background information

This is an unfortunate situation that has arisen, but which must be dealt with immediately. Behaviour that may be considered discriminatory, or disrespectful, is a serious act of professional misconduct. It is not enough in this situation to simply recognise events taking place. You will have an obligation to take action to bring about active steps to stop this behaviour. In all of these situations, you should work to clarify and confirm the situation with objective evidence that confirms your suspicions. This includes self-awareness and will be an impressive demonstration to the interviewers of your maturity and competence. We have used the **SCAM** approach in this station to first clarify the **S**cenario, place the events into an appropriate **C**ontext, **A**ppraise the evidence and then formulate an appropriate **M**anagement.

The GMC provides very clear and explicit guidance for issues in Good Medical Practice under 'Working with colleagues'.

1. Doctors must work effectively with colleagues from other health and social care disciplines
2. You must respect and value each person's skills and contributions

3. *You must tackle discrimination* where it arises, and encourage your colleagues to do the same

4. You must treat your colleagues fairly and with respect

5. You must not bully or harass them, or unfairly discriminate against them

6. *You should challenge the behaviour of colleagues* who do not meet this standard

7. You must get advice on these issues if you require it

You must actively advance equality and diversity by creating or maintaining a positive working environment – free from discrimination, bullying and harassment.

3.6 DRUNK CONSULTANT

'Your consultant arrives late to the morning ward round. You can clearly smell alcohol on his breath and you notice he is off-balance. On speaking to the first patient the consultant confuses them for a different patient on the ward and is ostensibly slurring his speech. How would you proceed?'

This is a precarious and potentially disastrous situation that must be acted on immediately. It is clear that the consultant has appeared inebriated on the ward round given his demeanour. He is clearly a danger to patients as well as himself, which is evident in his confusion of one of his patients. My primary concern at this stage would be to safeguard the patients as quickly and sensitively as possible. The easiest way to do this may be to contact another senior member of the team as soon as possible as they are more likely to have an impact on the consultant. If the registrar was not available or unable to help, I would then seek out another nearby consultant or senior staff nurse and inform them of the situation. It would be ideal to move the consultant away from the clinical area into a quiet, private room. This would protect the consultant from potentially harming himself in a clinical environment and also protects patients. If absolutely necessary the option of calling for security may need to be explored. Once this was organised, I would ensure an appropriate member of staff was with the consultant to prevent them placing themselves in a similar situation and then review the patients acutely affected. The patient who was being attended might have been distressed by the episode, and it would be important to reassure them. I would also identify any management plans, instructions or actions the consultant may have organised in his state and for the time being halt all such orders until a senior member of staff had reviewed them. Any emergency situations or orders I would bring to the immediate attention of the senior registrar, or if required, consultant on an appropriate team. It would be important to organise a suitable replacement to continue the care of the outstanding patients. This may be the senior registrar who may present any worrying or complicated patients and their management plans to a senior consultant. Following these actions, suitable arrangements would need to be made for the safe transport of the consultant home. An independent report should be written with accounts taken from all members involved. This may then be taken forward by the head of the surgery department, clinical/medical director or even the GMC. The consultant should be given supportive services with the aim of identifying any issues that may have caused this incident, and list steps taken to avoid this occurrence.

Background information

This is a popular question and in the past, it has revolved around a drunk consultant on a ward round, but variations include an inebriated consultant in the theatre or in the clinic. The question addresses your ability to act decisively with tact with the patient at the centre of your concern. The GMC guidance for this topic states:

1. All doctors have a duty to raise concerns when patient safety or care is compromised by colleagues.
2. Staff should be able to raise concerns in an open and safe environment.
3. You may be reluctant to report a concern for a number of reasons. For example, because you fear that nothing will be done or that raising your concern may cause problems for colleagues, have a negative effect on working relationships, have a negative effect on your career, or result in a complaint about you.
4. However, you have a duty to put patients' interests first and act to protect them, which overrides personal and professional loyalties.

5. The law provides legal protection against victimisation or dismissal for individuals who reveal information to raise genuine concerns and expose malpractice in the workplace

6. You do not need to wait for proof – you will be able to justify raising a concern if you do so honestly, on the basis of reasonable belief and through appropriate channels, even if you are mistaken

7. You must follow the procedure where you work for reporting near misses and incidents. This is because routinely identifying incidents or near misses at an early stage, can allow issues to be tackled, problems to be put right and lessons to be learnt.

3.7 LEADERSHIP AND MANAGEMENT

Leadership in the NHS

It is helpful to understand the principles behind good leadership and applying these in clinical practice. In more advanced interviews for registrar training numbers and consultant posts you are more likely to be pressed about your ability to lead a team. In the core surgical training interview, you are more likely to be asked more generic questions about what makes a good leader.

'What is the importance of self-analysis as a leader?'

Identifying traits in oneself is an important facet of leadership. Identifying important values and principles, as well as prejudices and shortcomings, are all essential in refining the ability to lead a team effectively and fairly. My own principles may differ widely with those of the team I am working with and it is therefore important to understand what impact this may have in my decision making, as well as behaviour. It would be essential through self-analysis to identify the strengths, weaknesses and limitations I have in order to elicit the most effective, competent and safe performance I could deliver. This is reflected in 360-degree feedback not only from peers, but also from a self multi-source feedback tool, which is important.

'What are the important factors in managing yourself?'

There is a high degree of organisation that is needed to ensure that clinical commitments, as well as personal responsibilities, are met. This includes being reliable and realistic when committing to responsibilities and ensuring these are completed to a high standard on a consistent basis. Flexibility that allows me to work around the needs of others, as well as planning for unexpected events such as emergencies, is also an important aspect of self-management. The clinical environment can be a stressful workplace and controlling my emotions and possible frustrations is vital to ensure a professional and conducive working practice. I would always ensure my behaviour and conduct towards others remained of the highest professional and respectable level, which requires self-control, particularly in stressful situations. This is particularly important when there is a conflict in decisions. Finally, managing workloads in the clinical, academic and extra-curricular domains is essential in order to ensure that on a personal level I do not compromise my own health while achieving my goals.

'Can you give examples of demonstrating integrity as a leader?'

Maintaining integrity as a leader includes upholding important professional ethics and values, and respecting the same for others taking into account their cultural and religious beliefs. Examples of this would include taking on responsibility as a core surgical trainee, and managing the foundation year 1 and year 2 members of the team. I would ensure there was a fair distribution of work across each member, including myself, and that no preference is given to any single trainee, and that I hold myself to the same values that I would expect from the junior team members. In episodes of dangerous or incompetent practice, I would not hesitate to clarify and then take appropriate actions to raise this to the appropriate person who can take action. Finally, being open to constructive advice and criticism in order to further my own competence and practice is important, and I would ensure I would ask for advice or admit to areas where I feel less confident or capable.

3.8 MANAGING STRESS

'What methods do you use or consider in order to manage your stress?'

There are various methods I use to manage my levels of stress, which is inevitable when working in surgery – but is not necessarily a bad or harmful thing if well controlled. Identifying when stress becomes detrimental rather than a driving or motivational factor is important, and I often speak to my colleagues in the first instance as a way of releasing or diffusing tension. This is helpful as voicing my thoughts can help identify and acknowledge difficult emotions regarding scenarios and situations in clinical practice. I often find that poor time management leads to stressful situations and therefore I have highlighted this through reflective practice. I have attended a time management course and also become more organised in setting realistic and achievable targets. It is easy to become engrossed in academic and clinical commitments, therefore I have invested time in personal growth away from the working environment, such as sport and religious activities. Other methods that are helpful that can be considered is spending more time with family and friends, which is often the best form of stress relief and a welcome break from work-related activities and discussions. Having a mentor at work is an invaluable tool that is increasing in popularity, with many courses available now that offer mentoring as well as teaching you to become a mentor yourself.

'How would you recognise a stressed colleague?'

Overwhelmed or stressed colleagues often demonstrate similar behaviours and traits as depressed individuals, and there are the outward signs I would look for. These would include a reduced interest or pleasure in activities, chronic feelings of tiredness or lack of energy and a poor diet that may include poor eating or over-eating. These are cardinal symptoms that an individual is suffering more than the baseline level of stress that can be considered normal. I would be particularly concerned if an individual showed clear signs of depression which can occur in acute, severe episodes of stress or constant, persistent stressful situations. These would include, among others, wanting to hurt yourself or not seeing any option other than being better off dead, feelings of hopelessness, poor concentration and extreme sleep disturbance.

'How can you prevent stress?'

Doctors are notorious for being the worst patients. There is considerable stigma around seeking help for work-related problems. This can arise from a multitude of reasons, including the fear of seeking help, or discussions not remaining confidential. In a hospital full of doctors, identifying oneself succumbing to stress can be an embarrassing and humiliating demonstration that is not always easy to overcome. I would therefore work on identifying signs of stress within myself and then act early on addressing the issues, for my own benefit as well as that of patients. I would work on any health issues that may arise as early as possible, and also seek help at work if this is the source of stress. Ignoring problems is often the most causative factor leading to stress and a deterioration in performance and health.

3.9 MENTAL CAPACITY ACT

You may be given scenarios featuring patients with mental health problems who lack capacity. We have outlined information next in a question and answer format to help you understand the principles of the Mental Capacity Act. You are unlikely to be asked in-depth detail about the act itself, but it is essential you understand it in order to apply it to a given scenario.

'What is the Mental Capacity Act?'

The Mental Capacity Act is an essential model that provides protection for individuals who are no longer able to make their own decisions. The act extends from assessing a person's ability to make a decision to providing care givers with the ability to make decisions on behalf of the person; also, it includes important safeguards for protection. The act is there to ensure – in the unfortunate situation that a person loses the ability to make their own decisions – that provisions are made which are in the patient's best interest, with the least impact on their rights.

'Who does the Mental Capacity Act apply to?'

The Mental Capacity Act defines a person who has suffered 'an impairment of, or a disturbance in the functioning of, the mind or brain'. This may be reversible to permanent, and in both situations the act protects the best interest of the affected patient. A patient is always presumed to have capacity until all efforts to aid them in making their own decision have been exhausted. A patient who is detained under the Mental Health Act is not automatically deemed to have lost capacity.

'What are the principles of the Mental Capacity Act?'

The principles of the mental capacity act can be best summarised by the various sections that outline the act itself. These include:

- Section 1(2) A person is assumed to have the capacity to make their decision until this is categorically proven to not be the case.
- Section 1(3) Any person who is being considered under the Mental Capacity Act should first be helped in every way to make their own decision
- Section 1(4) A person has every right to make a decision which may seem unwise to others. A decision the person makes that is not in their own best interest but one they have made themselves does not equate to a lack of capacity.
- Section 1(5) If a person is deemed to lack capacity then an action performed under the mental capacity act must only be in the best interest of the person.
- Section 1(6) Any action performed under the mental capacity act must be the least restrictive action possible.

Section 2 of the mental capacity act defines what lack of capacity means, whilst Section 3 outlines how to assess a person's capacity.

'What are the deprivation of liberty safeguards?'

Part 2 of the Mental Health Act of 2007 made amendments to the original 2005 act. This included safeguards if a person was to be deprived of their liberty. This is the result of a case labelled after the hospital 'Bournewood'. This dealt with a clash between depriving the liberty of a person under the Mental Health Act without breaching the European Convention on Human Rights. The amendments allowed lawful restrictions on the deprivation of liberty of people lacking capacity. These include:

- *Section 4A*: A person may be deprived of their liberty if this is to provide life-sustaining treatment.
- *Section 4B*: A person may be deprived of their liberty if this is secondary to a decision in court or schedule A1 (residents in hospitals and care homes).

'What legal protection does a decision maker have?'

Section 5 of the Mental Capacity Act provides care givers and decision makers for a person with capacity legal protection as long as they establish the person falls under the remit of the Mental Capacity Act and their decisions are in the persons best interest. Section 6 allows for appropriate physical restraint, in order to prevent harm, to a person under the act. This must be appropriate to the situation and cannot be used as a deprivation of liberty. Section 44 makes it strictly illegal to neglect or otherwise harm a person under the Mental Capacity Act. The court of protection oversees actions performed under the Mental Capacity Act and resolve any disputes. It wields the same power as the high court.

'What are deputies?'

If a person under the Mental Capacity Act does not have a lasting power of attorney, a substitute can be provided by the courts and are known as 'deputies'. They are able to make decisions for the best interest of the person with regards to health, wealth and finances. This can be a family member or close friend. The spouse does not have a legal right to act as a deputy. The court may also appoint an independent member who is outside of the family if more complex matters arise.

3.10 MID STAFFORDSHIRE ENQUIRY

The Mid Staffordshire enquiry represents an important series of failings that should be understood by every working clinician and is an area of discussion that may occur in the management station of the core surgical interview. Patients experienced appalling conditions and every doctor should be aware of this enquiry so that patients may never be subjected to this again. We have provided a summary of the important details of the enquiry in a series of question and answers to dually aid familiarisation with the enquiry as well as with the potential questions that may be asked.

'What is the background to the Mid Staffordshire Enquiry?'

The Mid Staffordshire enquiry is the investigation of the Mid Staffordshire NHS Foundation Trust which serves the population of Stafford. There were multiple and repeated instances where the delivery of service fell well below the acceptable, most basic human standard of care. These events occurred primarily between 2005 and 2008. The investigation was sparked from the onslaught of complaints from patients and their close family and friends for the appalling treatment that they had experienced. These complaints were largely ignored, or not taken seriously, by the trust board of the hospital leading to inadequate action at the time of the events. The multiple safety nets, checks, regulations and groups that are designed to highlight and prevent falls in acceptable standards of care all failed to detect or act on the events for a number of years. Importantly, the review and the enquiry highlights an attitude and culture within the hospital that accepted the poor quality of care and developed a tolerance for allowing such standards to continue.

'How bad were the events that occurred at the hospital?'

The enquiry highlighted the following examples of patient care and treatment:

1. Patients were allowed to remain in their own soiled bed clothes for prolonged periods of time.
2. Repeated requests by patients to assist them in attending the toilet were ignored.
3. Patients who were unable to feed themselves were not given assistance.
4. Water was not easily reachable by patients.
5. The enquiry quotes the wards and toilet facilities to have been left in a 'filthy condition'.
6. Patients' right to dignity and privacy, even following a death, were not respected.
7. Triage of patients in A/E was undertaken by inappropriate staff who did not have the required level of training.
8. Staff demonstrated a cold and 'callous' attitude that was indifferent to their level of suffering with no empathy to the conditions patients were left in through no fault of their own (i.e., no fault of the patients).
9. Multiple other failings that spanned across patient safety, diagnosis, investigation and management. As well as in infection control, discharge and documentation.
10. The events had occurred whilst the hospital had been raised to 'Foundation Trust' level.

'What were the solutions offered following the enquiry?'

i. A strong emphasis on changing the institutional culture that places the patient first and foremost. Producing a recognisable standard of care that was acceptable to staff and patient with a zero-tolerance attitude if that level was breached.

ii. Open and honest evidence regarding any matters of concerns within the hospital.

iii. A sense of accountability and responsibility for anyone involved in the care of a patient with appropriate recruitment of staff involved in healthcare.

iv. Develop methods of measuring and ensuring the compliance and adherence to the aforementioned standards across all individuals, teams, units and organisations.

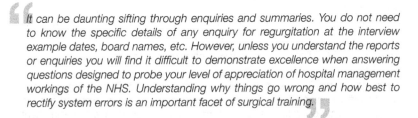

It can be daunting sifting through enquiries and summaries. You do not need to know the specific details of any enquiry for regurgitation at the interview example dates, board names, etc. However, unless you understand the reports or enquiries you will find it difficult to demonstrate excellence when answering questions designed to probe your level of appreciation of hospital management workings of the NHS. Understanding why things go wrong and how best to rectify system errors is an important facet of surgical training.

Potential questions that may arise from this topic:

1. How would you deal with a situation where a colleague is mistreating a patient?
2. How would you raise a concern about hospital standards?
3. What examples do you know of public enquiries?
4. What are the potential reasons for a lapse in patient care?
5. Who is responsible for dealing with a hospital complaint?
6. How can a patient, family member or friend raise a concern or complaint in hospital?
7. Who would you seek first if you have concerns about a:
   a. Nurse
   b. Doctor
   c. Registrar
   d. Consultant

3.11 NCEPOD

'What is NCEPOD?'

The National Confidential Enquiry into Perioperative Deaths (NCEPOD) is a government supported initiative that helps to maintain and improve upon the care of patients in all medical and surgical specialties. NCEPOD reports on mortalities that occur following surgery with the aim of evaluating the events and identifying areas of improvement. It does this by performing confidential surveys, audits and research of patient care, with publication of its findings for the benefit of the public and all healthcare professionals.

An example of NCEPOD findings and suggestions from past reports include:

1. Highlighting the increased complication rate and mortality from operations conducted outside normal working hours. Surgical practice has changed as a result of this with night operations strictly reserved for emergency cases. Every patient is assessed according to a given standard for the urgency of their procedure, and an emergency list formulated accordingly.

2. Surgeons and anaesthetists should be involved in regular multidisciplinary audits and meetings. The aim of these meetings is to identify changes in the systems of practice that will prevent further mistakes or near misses from occurring, and help safeguard patients.

3. Central venous pressure management and interpretation is an area of weakness for doctors and nurses. National and local training programmes have been recommended to aid expertise, particularly in intensive care and high dependency units.

4. Review of patients suffering from cancer. NCEPOD demonstrated that the majority of patients with cancer dying within 30 days of an operation are admitted as an emergency or urgently. There is not a more rapid referral pathway to an appropriate surgeon with oncology interest or a multidisciplinary team, medical oncologist or specialist cancer nurse when indicated.

'How does NCEPOD work?'

NCEPOD originated from a pilot study performed by Lunn and Mushin in 1982, which examined the anaesthesia-related mortality across several regions in the United Kingdom. The aim of the study was to improve the safety and quality of anaesthetic practice through the evaluation of perioperative patient data. An important aspect of this included creating a standard of care as part of the study. Following the study, the Confidential Enquiry into Perioperative Deaths (CEPOD) was established to examine both surgical and anaesthetic patients with NCEPOD in 1988 to cover all specialities in medicine.

There are not always recognised standards of care for NCEPOD to use to compare with current practice. Unlike an audit, where the current standard is compared to a given gold standard, NCEPOD often assesses what standard a particular service is achieving.

NCEPOD employs staff to visit hospitals and give presentations at appropriate meetings (e.g., audit days). If a concerning case is identified by NCEPOD, it is referred to the medical director of the Trust as well as to the consultants involved with the patient.

'What is the NCEPOD classification of intervention?'

In order to determine the level of urgency of an operation or procedure, NCEPOD initially used a 4 code system of classification which included 'Emergency', 'Urgent', 'Scheduled' and 'Elective'. This has now been changed to 'Immediate', 'Urgent', 'Expedited' and 'Elective'.

1. *Immediate*: An intervention that is organ-, limb- or life-saving. The condition may be of such severity that resuscitation occurs in tandem with the intervention. Patients are typically operated on within minutes of making a decision.

2. *Urgent*: An intervention or procedure to treat the acute occurrence or deterioration of an organ, limb or a life-threatening condition. This also includes other conditions such as fracture fixation. Patients are typically operated on within hours of making a decision.

3. *Expedited*: The patient qualifies for early treatment for a condition that does not pose an immediate risk to organ, limb or life. Patients are typically operated within days of making a decision.

4. *Elective*: Non-emergency intervention that can be planned to suit the patient and hospital as part of a routine hospital admission.

It would be reasonable to identify other major categories and several subcategories to those given previously, however, the classification is also designed to be as simple and user-friendly as possible. The consultant performing the procedure typically designates the intervention category. This is recorded in the theatre management system, as well as in the patients' case notes.

'What are the advantages of the NCEPOD classification?'

1. The allocation of theatres and procedure lists is made easier and more streamlined, especially for acute same-day decision making.

2. As supported by studies, patients are operated on within a time frame that is appropriate for the condition they have presented with and where appropriately escalated in priority.

3. Only appropriate out-of-hours procedures are performed.

NCEPOD revised classification of operation

Description	Target time to theatre	Expected location	Example scenarios	Typical procedures	Description	Target time to theatre
Immediate (A) lifesaving or (B) limb- or organ-saving intervention. Resuscitation simultaneous with surgical treatment	Within minutes of decision to operate	Next available operating theatre – 'break-in' to existing lists if required	1. Ruptured aortic aneurysm; 2. Major trauma to abdomen or thorax; 3. Fracture with major neurovascular deficit; 4. Compartment syndrome. Acute myocardial infarction	1. Repair of ruptured aortic aneurysm; 2. Laparotomy/thoracotomy for control of haemorrhage; 3. Fasciotomy; 4. Coronary angioplasty	Immediate (A) lifesaving; or (B) limb- or organ-saving intervention. Resuscitation simultaneous with surgical treatment	Within minutes of decision to operate
Acute onset or deterioration of conditions that threaten life, limb or organ survival; fixation of fractures; relief of distressing symptoms.	Within hours of decision to operate and normally once resuscitation completed	Daytime 'emergency' list or out-of-hours emergency theatre (including at night)	1. Compound fracture; 2. Perforated bowel with peritonitis; 3. Critical organ or limb ischaemia; 4. Acute coronary syndrome; 5. Perforating eye injuries	1. Debridement plus fixation of fracture; 2. Laparotomy for perforation; 3. Coronary angioplasty	Acute onset or deterioration of conditions that threaten life, limb or organ survival; Fixation of fractures; Relief of distressing symptoms.	Within hours of decision to operate and normally once resuscitation completed
Stable patient requiring early intervention for a condition that is not an immediate threat to life, limb or organ survival	Within days of decision to operate	Elective list which has 'spare' capacity or Daytime 'emergency' list (not at night)	1. Tendon and nerve injuries; 2. Stable & non-septic patients for wide range of surgical procedures; 3. Retinal detachment	1. Repair of tendon and nerve injuries; 2. Excision of tumour with potential to bleed or obstruct; 3. Coronary angioplasty	Stable patient requiring early intervention for a condition that is not an immediate threat to life, limb or organ survival	Within days of decision to operate
Surgical procedure planned or booked in advance of routine admission to hospital	Planned	Elective theatre list booked & planned prior to admission	Encompasses all conditions not classified as immediate, urgent or expedited.	1. Elective AAA repair; 2. Laparoscopic cholecystectomy; 3. Varicose vein surgery; 4. Joint replacement; 5. Coronary angioplasty	Surgical procedure planned or booked in advance of routine admission to hospital	Planned

3.12 NURSE PRACTITIONER

'What is a nurse practitioner in surgery?'

A nurse practitioner in surgery, or otherwise known as a surgical care practitioner, is defined by the National Curriculum Framework for Surgical Care Practitioners as: '... a non-medical practitioner, working in clinical practice as a member of the extended surgical team, who performs surgical intervention, preoperative and postoperative care under the direction and supervision of a consultant surgeon'.

'Do we need nurse practitioners?'

A surgical trainee at any level up to and including a consultant would agree that, alongside falling specialist registrar numbers and reduced junior team members, the demands of the population from a surgical perspective will only continue to grow. Even fully staffed, surgical teams at any given moment face an uphill struggle to meet the service provision requirements of the surgical department. With mounting social and policy pressure to expedite patient consultation, reduce waiting times and allow prompt treatment, well trained and experienced surgical care practitioners would seem a welcome and gratefully accepted service.

'What roles could nurse practitioners fulfil in surgery?'

As part of the service provision needs of a surgical department, nurse practitioners can aid the preoperative assessment and preparation of patients for surgical intervention. This could include, but is not limited to, time-consuming tasks such as venepuncture, cannulation and results analysis under supervision. Studies have also shown that appropriate experienced nurse practitioners serve as competent technical assistants to an operating surgeon without compromising outcomes. Indeed, the first nurse practitioner in the United Kingdom was utilised to harvest the long saphenous vein for coronary artery bypass grafting. A sobering thought is despite competition and other problems, doctors have a structured training pathway with clear roles (e.g., foundation level, core trainee, specialist registrar and consultant). Nurses represent the vast majority of the NHS work force and operate at the front line of services with poor financial remuneration and limited promotional opportunities. The role of a nurse practitioner may therefore be a well overdue and necessary addition to structured nurse training.

'What are the advantages of a nurse practitioner in surgery?'

There are multiple potential benefits of a nurse practitioner service within surgery. Since they would not be bound by the same work shift patterns created by the European Working Time Directive (EWTD), they can fill the voids created by rotating surgical doctors at every level by being a constant and consistent member of the team. There is also a significant financial incentive, since the cost of training a nurse care practitioner is marginal compared to a doctor. Studies also support comparable productivity, quality of care and patient satisfaction. With ever-changing NHS structures, nurse practitioners represent a versatile general surgical asset with transferable skills that can easily mould into other roles if required, unlike senior trained staff that often invest significant time periods for a specific role.

'What are the potential concerns of having a nurse practitioner in surgery?'

Despite clear advantages to having a nurse practitioner to complement the surgical team there remain concerns and caveats to their presence. The most obvious is of course surgical exposure for junior and to a lesser extent senior trainees. It is a well-known fact that surgical trainees must often compete amongst themselves for elective and emergency theatre lists, which is compounded by the limitations of the EWTD. A nurse practitioner being trained operatively must directly compete with a junior surgical trainee to acquire basic surgical skills. One can also argue that nurse practitioners represent a short fix without addressing the original reason for their deployment – filling the gaps left by a shortage of doctors. Proponents for surgical care practitioners may argue their role as complementing the work of surgical trainees, and by performing more minor and routine operations, trainees remain free for more advanced procedures. This argument often does not stand since basic surgical training is dependent on repetition and mastering of basic, routine procedures so that basic skills can be transferred to more demanding operations. Also, a reduced period of surgical training must be matched by an increase in intensity and quality of surgical practice, which would be limited by sharing operations with non-trainees.

'Do nurse practitioners in surgery only affect junior trainees?'

Although the most obvious concern may be reduced surgical exposure for junior trainees, consultants are also likely to be affected since they are the most obvious choice for the supervision of a nurse practitioners with an operative role. The impact of this is not only a dilution in the operative opportunities for surgical trainees but also for senior training opportunities. Core surgical trainees and specialist registrars also undergo rigorous and regular assessments with clinical and educational supervisors to measure progress and competency. A similar assessment of nurse practitioners would be necessary to maintain a standardised and regulated training service.

'What impact would nurse practitioners have on patient care?'

As mentioned already, there are clear benefits to service provision with nurse practitioners employed in a surgical department. Patient surveys have made clear that they would wish to be clearly informed that their practitioner was not medically qualified, although trained adequately for the examination, investigation or intervention they may be offered by the nurse practitioner. Patients retain the right to request a preference for a medically qualified person, without any impact upon their healthcare experience.

3.13 REVALIDATION

What is revalidation? Revalidation was launched in 2012 as a demonstration and assurance to patients and employers that a licensed doctor remains fit to practice, and is considered current with the standards of healthcare. The GMC introduced licenses for all UK doctors in 2009, as a means of registration and a passport to practice medicine, regardless of position or seniority. Revalidation renews this licence in accordance to the principles outlined in Good Medical Practice, and is a legal requirement for UK doctors. Revalidation takes place every 5 years, alongside annual employer appraisal.

'What is the process of revalidation?'

1. All licensed doctors will liaise with an impartial individual who will act as their responsible officer (typically a senior doctor themselves).
2. Good Medical Practice is used to appraise and evaluate doctors on their core skills. For those in recognised training programmes this is undertaken through the Annual Review of Competence Progression (ARCP), and the responsible officer is the postgraduate dean of the deanery (now known as local education and training boards). All doctors must keep an updated portfolio that acts to support the core foundations provided in Good Medical Practice, based on their experience in the clinical environment.
3. The responsible officer uses this portfolio, alongside formal appraisals, to assess whether a doctor remains fit for practice and recommends them for revalidation to the GMC. The GMC uses this recommendation amongst other safeguards to grant revalidation where appropriate.

'What is the Good Medical Practice framework for revalidation?'

This consists of four domains that represent the standard of clinical practice, and against which appraisal and revalidation is based upon.

Domain 1 – Knowledge, skills, and performance

1.1 Maintain your professional performance

1.2 Apply knowledge and experience to practice

1.3 Ensure that all documentation (including clinical records) formally recording your work is clear, accurate and legible

Domain 2 – Safety and quality

2.1 Contribute to and comply with systems to protect patients

2.2 Respond to risks to safety

2.3 Protect patients and colleagues from any risk posed by your health

Domain 3 – Communication, partnership, and teamwork

3.1 Communicate effectively

3.2 Work constructively with colleagues and delegate effectively

3.3 Establish and maintain partnerships with patients

Domain 4 – Maintaining trust

    4.1 Show respect for patients

    4.2 Treat patients and colleagues fairly and without discrimination

    4.3 Act with honesty and integrity

'How would a model appraisal take place?'

Based on the NHS revalidation support team, a model appraisal would include:

1. A primary input that outlines what your work entails including your clinical responsibilities and all actions related to patient care (e.g., clinical, academic, educational and extracurricular)

2. A secondary input would include supporting information for continuing professional development, quality improvement activity, significant events, feedback from colleagues and patients, compliments and complaints

3. A review of the personal development plan should also be undertaken with analysis of objectives and how these have been fulfilled with a discussion of career goals and ambitions. There must also be a discussion on clinical practice development and reflection

4. Each doctor must agree and accept the probity and health statements based on Good Medical Practice and be accountable for the information they provide to support their appraisal

5. The outcome of the appraisal is summarised under the four domains listed above. A revalidation decision is made based upon these statements and a new personal development plan.

3.14 SCREENING

Screening is a popular topic upon which discussions may occur and we advise you to familiarise yourself not only with the basic concepts, but also with more advanced areas to demonstrate your excellence and calibre. We have outlined information next in a question and answer format.

'What is screening?'

A screening programme is a method of analysing individuals who are not known to have the disease that is being investigated. The purpose of this is to identify a given disease or a precursor that may lead to a given disease early. This allows for preventative measures to be taken for disease prevention, delay its progression or improve its prognosis.

'What is a good screening programme?'

A good screening programme should involve a number of traits in order for it to be successfully integrated and employed for the general population. Screening should identify a disease which if detected early, can lead to an improved prognosis. This may also apply to risk factors which are proven to cause a given disease pathology. The WHO criteria for a screening programme are as follows:

1. The disease should be an important health problem
2. There should be a well-recognised pre-clinical stage to the disease including symptoms and infectious state
3. The natural history of the disease should be well understood including risk factors, disease markers and latent periods, and so forth
4. There should be a significant time period between objective signs of the disease and development into overt pathology
5. There should be a diagnostic test available to confirm disease status
6. The validity of the screening programme should have high sensitivity and specificity
7. The screening should be simple to perform, safe and acceptable in its methods
8. The screening methods should be reliable
9. The disease should have adequate treatment options that are effective and safe
10. Facilities should be suitable to provide screening measures
11. The programme should be economically viable
12. The programme should be sustainable

'What are the limitations of screening?'

Despite a large number of prerequisites for screening programmes no initiative, investigation or test is 100% reliable. This therefore creates the potential of doing harm to patients who may enter a programme with no disease, and undergo considerable distress and anxiety which may have been avoided. There must therefore be enough evidence to justify a screening programme against the multiple potential harms that can be caused.

'What is validity?'

The validity of any test can be measured by its ability to determine those patients with a condition and those without. In order to evaluate the validity of an investigation, the true disease status must be obtainable, usually through a gold standard measure.

'What is sensitivity and specificity?'

This can be best described using the following model:

Disease Status (as per gold standard)

		Diseased	Not diseased	
Test Result	Positive:	a	b	a + b
	Negative:	c	d	c + d
		a + c	b + d	

Sensitivity: This describes the test's ability to highlight those patients who have the disease:

$$\text{Sensitivity} = a/(a + c)$$

Specificity: This describes the test's ability to highlight those patients who do not have the disease:

$$\text{Specificity} = d/(b + d)$$

'What is a positive and negative predictive value?'

The positive predictive value represents how likely it is that a patient (which has tested positive) actually has the disease.

$$\text{Positive predictive value} = a/(a + b)$$

The negative predictive value represents how likely it is that a patient (which has tested negative) does not actually have the disease.

$$\text{Negative predictive value} = a/(a + b)$$

'What are the approaches to screening?'

Screening may be systematically conducted or be opportunistic. In both methods, patients may be screened as part of a mass exercise or a subselection of patients who are at an increased risk of the disease in question.

'What are the major screening programmes in the United Kingdom?'

Antenatal screening: Syphilis, HIV, hepatitis B, rubella, chromosome abnormalities, fetal growth, etc.

Neonatal and childhood: Phenylketonuria, congenital hip dislocation, hypothyroidism, haemoglobinopathies and sickle cell disease (tend to be concentrated in areas of high prevalence), hearing and development.

Cancer: Breast and cervical cancer in women, bowel cancer for all men and women aged between 60 and 69.

Infections: Chlamdyia in the under 25-years-old population. Hepatitis B screening is mandatory for anyone involved in healthcare. Sexual health clinics also offer HIV screening as an optional service.

Cardiovascular disease: Screening is conducted for blood pressure, high cholesterol and diabetes.

Criteria for Screening (based on WHO criteria)

1. Disease
2. Important health problem
3. Well recognized pre-clinical stage
4. Natural history understood
5. Long period between first signs and overt disease
6. Diagnostic test
7. Valid (sensitive and specific)
8. Simple and cheap
9. Safe and acceptable
10. Reliable
11. Diagnosis and treatment
12. Facilities are adequate
13. Effective, acceptable and safe treatment available
14. Cost effective
15. Sustainable

Evaluating screening programmes

Even after a suitable screening tool is made available, there are a number of important factors that still must be considered:

Feasibility: This describes the ease with which a population can be screened using the test, its acceptability and whether resources are available to follow-up the results of the screening (e.g., investigations).

Effectiveness: This is measured by the outcomes of a screening programme once it is executed, and is difficult to assess due to various types of bias; among others, these include:

Selection bias: Participants of screening programmes are generally different from those that do not volunteer

Lead time bias: Here, a screening programme correctly identifies a disease and gives the impression that survival has been extended due to early recognition. However, such patients would have been identified later due to various reasons (manifestation of disease, symptoms, signs, etc.). The screening programme therefore does not actually improve survival or prognosis, but simply identifies the disease earlier.

Cost

The cost effectiveness of a screening programme is always an important and often decisive factor. This is not only related to the screening initiative itself, but must also consider the following investigations and management of the condition once correctly identified. The costs of a screening programme are often balanced against treating those patients who present later with often more advanced and complicated disease.

Ethical considerations

A screening population is usually fit and healthy from their own perspective and therefore would not normally have requested for the test themselves. Therefore, the impact that a screening investigation has on an individual is of utmost importance with important consequences such as:

1. The patient may undergo needless anxiety and emotional trauma from a false positive result
2. Screening investigations may have inherent risks themselves
3. False negative results can be falsely reassuring

3.15 STATISTICS A-Z

You may be asked to expand on basic statistical terms in the interview, or discuss scenarios that include some basic statistical terminology. We have compiled an A-Z list of terms to ensure you are familiar with these. You will not be asked to critique a paper itself, perform or interpret statistics, however knowledge and use of these terms will instantly set you well apart from other candidates. You may be asked to expand on the methodology section of any publications in the portfolio station, and this section is therefore useful for this purpose also.

Attributable risk

The attributable risk represents the risk that is due to the exposure being investigated. It demonstrates how much greater the frequency of a disease in an exposure group is compared to an unexposed. This importantly assumes that the exposure is causal for a disease.

Attributable risk = Incidence in the exposed - Incidence in the unexposed

Example: If 30 out of 100 smokers contracted lung cancer in a set period of time and these patients were compared to 10 non-smokers out of 100 who also had lung cancer we can calculate the relative risk (see next) and the attributable risk:

Relative risk: $30/10 = 3$

Attributable risk: $(30–10)/100 = 20$ per 100. This can be shown as an express fraction by $20/30 = 66\%$

What this means is that of the 30 patients in the smoking group that suffered lung cancer, 20 cases (i.e. 66%) can be attributed to smoking.

Case

A case must be clearly identified so that research can accurately identify the occurrences of this disease or condition in the population.

Case-control study

Study that recruits participants based on them having the outcome that is being measured (i.e., each participant must be a case). These tend to be rare diseases. Case-control studies can be used to explore exposure as a risk factor more common in individuals with a disease than without. The result of this study is therefore an **odds ratio** (the odds of having an exposure such as asbestos and suffering from the case e.g. mesothelioma, compared to the odds of being exposed to asbestos and not having mesothelioma.)

Cause

Often the driving force behind most studies and the question that they attempt to answer, for example, does HRT therapy cause increased DVT risk in patients? Does electromagnetic exposure cause leukaemia in children? And so forth. Research studies attempt to disprove the alternative explanations and confounding factors for a given question. If this is successful, then causation can be proved.

Chi-squared test

This is a statistical test that shows whether two proportions are similar to each other through significance. For example, is a proportion of patients with liver cirrhosis who drink alcohol significantly different to a proportion of patients with liver cirrhosis who do not. The lower the value, the less likely such groups are of being similar to each other, and there is therefore a significant difference.

Cohort study

Participants are recruited to a cohort study if they have been exposed to a stimulant of interest. They are then followed over a period of time and compared to a matched, non-exposed group. The outcome from this is a relative risk.

Confidence interval

(95%) confidence intervals are a range of values within which the true value is likely to be contained. For example, a (95%) confidence interval from A to B based on relative risk would in 95% of cases contain the true relative risk between values A and B. If the interval between A and B does not include the value 1 for relative risk and odds ratio, then the null hypothesis (see later) is often rejected. If the interval does not include 0 instead of 1 for specific measures, such as blood pressure, then again, the null hypothesis is rejected (this is further explained under null hypothesis).

Confounding

A confounding factor can mask reasonable, alternative explanations that favour the null hypothesis to be correct, and must be accounted for as much as possible in order to prove causality. Such factors may include age, sex, smoking, social backgrounds, and so on.

Control

This is in contrast to a case, and is a participant who does not have the outcome of interest, nor is receiving the intervention or treatment being analysed.

Incidence

This is the number of new cases that occur over a defined period of time in a defined population.

Matching

This is an important and essential method that attempts to remove confounding factors such as age and sex in a case-control study. Control participants are recruited based on their similarity to the case participants while not having the outcome of interest.

Null hypothesis

The null hypothesis is the focus for statistical tests to disprove in a research study. The null hypothesis states that there is no difference between the two groups a researcher is investigating. If the groups were comparing rates the null hypothesis would imply that the rate of group A is equal to group B, that is 1. In a case-control study, the odds ratio in group A would equal group B, again equalling 1. This is why in a confidence interval for relative risk or odds ratio, the null hypothesis can be rejected if the interval does not include 1. For explicit variables such blood pressure and cholesterol levels, the null hypothesis would state that the value in group A is equal to the value in group B, hence $A - B = 0$. Therefore, the null hypothesis is rejected if the confidence interval does not include 0.

Odds and Odds ratio

Odds: This is an alternative term for probability expressed as:

$$Odds = probability/(1 - probability)$$

Odds ratio: The odds ratio simply divides the odds value in one group with the other odds of exposure in the case group divided by the odds of exposure in the control group. The odds ratio is used in case-control studies rather than the relative risk. A ratio greater than 1 implies that the exposure is more likely in the case group compared to the control group, and vice versa for a ratio less than 1.

Prevalence

This is the total number of cases in a defined population over a defined period of time. The same value obtained from a specific point in time rather than period is the 'point prevalence'. Importantly, the prevalence includes both new and old cases in contrast to incidence.

P-Value

The p-value is the probability of achieving the outcome of interest if the null hypothesis is shown to be true. The smaller the p-value (e.g., $p < 0.05$), the easier it is to reject the null hypothesis and accept the results of the study as being significant and not due to chance and other confounding factors.

Risk

From an epidemiological perspective, risk implies the chance or probability that an individual has of getting the outcome of interest.

Relative risk

The relative risk measures the degree of association between an exposure and disease. It is the ratio of the incidence rate in an exposure group, compared to the incidence rate in a non-exposed group.

Relative risk = incidence in exposed group/incidence in non-exposed group

A relative risk of 1 indicates that there is no association between exposure and disease state, a value that exceeds 1 supports an association whilst a value less than 1 suggests the exposure is protective against the disease state.

3.16 STERILISATION

'What is sterilisation?'

It is a method by which organisms, typically on surgical instruments, can be eradicated for reuse in patients. Multiple methods can be employed depending on the type of instrument and the level of sterilisation, disinfection or cleaning that is required.

Method	Activity	Example	Instrument
Sterilisation			
High temperature	All organisms including bacterial spores are eradicated	Steam and dry heat	Most reusable surgical instruments
Low temperature	All organisms including bacterial spores are eradicated	ETO gas and hydrogen peroxide gas	Most reusable surgical instruments
Liquid immersion	All organisms including bacterial spores are eradicated	Chemical sterilants	Most reusable surgical instruments
Autoclaving	All organisms including bacterial spores are eradicated	High pressure steam is used typically at 134°C for 3 minutes)	Most reusable surgical instruments, not suitable for fragile items
Glutaraldehyde solution (2%)	All organisms including bacterial spores are eradicated	Colourless oily liquid	Endoscopes and selected laparoscopic instruments. Staff are at risk of developing allergies hence limiting more wide usage
Ethylene oxide	All organisms including bacterial spores are eradicated	3% mixture of gas with carbon dioxide	Packaged heat sensitive equipment e.g., sutures
Gamma irradiation	All organisms including bacterial spores are eradicated	Gamma rays emitted from radioactive substance such as cobalt 60 or caesium 137	Heat tolerant instruments e.g., catheters and syringes

'What is disinfection?'

Disinfection differs from sterilisation in that it is far less efficacious, and not all viral and bacterial spore organisms are destroyed.

Method	Activity	Example	Instrument/other use
Disinfection			
Heat automated	All organisms except high numbers of bacterial spores	Pasteurization	Heat-tolerant surgical instruments
Liquid immersion	All organisms except high numbers of bacterial spores	Chemical sterilants	GI endoscopes and bronchoscopes
Liquid contact	Vegetative bacteria, mycobacteria, most viruses, and most fungi but not bacterial spores	EPA-registered hospital disinfectants	Blood-pressure cuffs, surfaces such as bedside tables, etc.
Skin			
Alcohol	Effective against bacteria but not against fungi or spores	Alcohol	Wards
Chlorhexidine	Effective against bacteria	Chlorhexidine	Theatre
Iodine	All organisms including bacterial spores are eradicated.	Iodine	Theatre

3.17 SEPSIS

'What is sepsis and septic shock?'

The International Guidelines for Management of Severe Sepsis and Septic Shock defines septic shock as 'hypotension persisting after initial fluid challenge or blood lactate concentration $\geq$4 mmol/L'. The signs of sepsis include: 'Fever, chills, hypothermia, leukocytosis, left shift of neutrophils, neutropenia, and the development of otherwise unexplained organ dysfunction (e.g., renal failure or signs of haemodynamic compromise) are specific indications for obtaining blood for culture. Blood cultures should be taken as soon as possible after the onset of fever or chills'.

'What are the sepsis six steps?'

The sepsis six steps double the survival chances of the patient, and include:

1. Administer high flow oxygen
2. Take blood cultures
3. Give broad spectrum antibiotics
4. Give intravenous fluid challenges
5. Measure serum lactate and haemoglobin
6. Measure accurate hourly urine output

'How can the aetiology of sepsis be established?'

1. Blood cultures may be obtained as long as they do not delay the initiation of antibiotic treatment by more than 45 mins. Current recommendations are that a minimum of two sets of blood cultures (aerobic and anaerobic) should be obtained prior to the initiation of treatment. Of the two blood cultures taken, one should be drawn percutaneously and one drawn through each vascular access device, unless these devices have been placed within 48 hours
2. Imaging studies are also recommended to be performed promptly to confirm a potential source of infection.

'Following a diagnosis of sepsis what should be completed within the first 3 hours?'

1. Measure lactate level from an arterial or venous source
2. Obtain two or more blood cultures prior to antibiotic administration
3. Administer broad spectrum antibiotics
4. Administer 30 mL/kg crystalloid for hypotension or lactate $\geq$4 mmol/L

'Following a diagnosis of sepsis what should be completed within 6 hours?'

1. Apply vasopressors (for hypotension that does not respond to initial fluid resuscitation) to maintain a mean arterial pressure (MAP) $\geq$65 mm Hg
2. In the event of persistent arterial hypotension despite volume resuscitation (septic shock) or initial lactate $\geq$4 mmol/L

3. Measure central venous pressure (CVP)
4. Measure central venous oxygen saturation (ScvO$_2$)
5. Re-measure lactate if initial lactate was elevated

'What are the goals in the first 6 hours of resuscitation for septic shock?'

1. The central venous pressure (CVP) should be maintained between 8–12 mm Hg
2. The mean arterial pressure (MAP) should be maintained at $\geq$ 65 mm Hg
3. The urine output should be $\geq$0.5 mL/kg/hr
4. Central venous (superior vena cava) oxygen saturation should be 70% (mixed venous oxygen saturation at 65%)
5. In patients with elevated lactate levels, these should be specifically targeted during resuscitation and normalized

'What antibiotics should be given?'

The choice between antibiotics is best decided by the most likely pathogens prevalent at the hospital alongside patient-specific knowledge including but not limited to past medical history, drug intolerances and current presenting condition. The regimen should be broad-spectrum and cover all likely pathogens, as the guidelines state 'there is little margin for error in critically ill patients'.

3.18 THE 'HOSPITAL AT NIGHT' PROJECT

The 'Hospital at Night' project is an initiative designed to tackle the issues raised by the European Working Time Directive to meet the service requirements needed during night time in the hospital. Rather than reflect the daytime working pattern – whereby each specialty has its own dedicated team – at night, when requirements are altered, a multi-disciplinary team is utilised for this purpose. Nursing staff and doctors cross-cover appropriate groups of patients, or across specialties, on the premise that generic transferable emergency skills can be employed across specialties – with secondary support available if more complex or specialist input is needed. An example of this would be a core surgical trainee who usually covers general surgery (a doctor covering multiple specialties) while on-call cross covering both general surgery, urology and orthopaedics when out of hours or at night. The duplication of multiple services is thus effectively tackled and ensures staff remain compliant with the EWTD.

An audit explored the demands of the hospital at night, and established the following:

- Many tasks performed by doctors could be distributed to non-medical personnel
- There was significant variation across specialties with regards to urgency or emergency demands, e.g., medical specialties generally had more ill patients requiring urgent or emergency services compared to surgery

As a result, there have been supportive programmes to help doctors working at night. This includes where possible:

- The use of nurse practitioners who can attend to more simple jobs, such as IV cannulation and fluid prescription, allowing doctors to remain more alert and focus their attention on patients who may require more input
- Medications and procedures are dealt with early in the daytime in order to reduce issues at night and when possible, alter the timing of interventions to minimise the workload for the night staff
- Reducing elective operating theatre slots to accommodate for emergency cases, hence reducing the risk of performing elective operations at night, due to delays caused by emergencies, when there is less support available
- The modified early warning system score (MEWS), or variations based on vital signs allows nursing staff to identify at-risk patients early, and escalate them to appropriate services. This is successfully employed both at night and daytime

3.19 WHO CHECKLIST

'What is the WHO checklist?'

The WHO checklist is a measure that streamlines the format of all operations such that the surgical team in the theatre follow a number of critical safety steps. The benefit of this is to reduce mistakes that could otherwise be avoided, and minimise the danger to surgical patients.

World Health Organization

SURGICAL SAFETY CHECKLIST (FIRST EDITION)

Before induction of anaesthesia ►►►►►►►► **Before skin incision** ►►►►►►►►►►►► **Before patient leaves operating room**

SIGN IN

- PATIENT HAS CONFIRMED
  - IDENTITY
  - SITE
  - PROCEDURE
  - CONSENT
- SITE MARKED/NOT APPLICABLE
- ANAESTHESIA SAFETY CHECK COMPLETED
- PULSE OXIMETER ON PATIENT AND FUNCTIONING

DOES PATIENT HAVE A:

KNOWN ALLERGY?
- NO
- YES

DIFFICULT AIRWAY/ASPIRATION RISK?
- NO
- YES, AND EQUIPMENT/ASSISTANCE AVAILABLE

RISK OF >500ML BLOOD LOSS (7ML/KG IN CHILDREN)?
- NO
- YES, AND ADEQUATE INTRAVENOUS ACCESS AND FLUIDS PLANNED

TIME OUT

- CONFIRM ALL TEAM MEMBERS HAVE INTRODUCED THEMSELVES BY NAME AND ROLE
- SURGEON, ANAESTHESIA PROFESSIONAL AND NURSE VERBALLY CONFIRM
  - PATIENT
  - SITE
  - PROCEDURE

ANTICIPATED CRITICAL EVENTS

- SURGEON REVIEWS: WHAT ARE THE CRITICAL OR UNEXPECTED STEPS, OPERATIVE DURATION, ANTICIPATED BLOOD LOSS?
- ANAESTHESIA TEAM REVIEWS: ARE THERE ANY PATIENT-SPECIFIC CONCERNS?
- NURSING TEAM REVIEWS: HAS STERILITY (INCLUDING INDICATOR RESULTS) BEEN CONFIRMED? ARE THERE EQUIPMENT ISSUES OR ANY CONCERNS?

HAS ANTIBIOTIC PROPHYLAXIS BEEN GIVEN WITHIN THE LAST 60 MINUTES?
- YES
- NOT APPLICABLE

IS ESSENTIAL IMAGING DISPLAYED?
- YES
- NOT APPLICABLE

SIGN OUT

- NURSE VERBALLY CONFIRMS WITH THE TEAM:
- THE NAME OF THE PROCEDURE RECORDED
- THAT INSTRUMENT, SPONGE AND NEEDLE COUNTS ARE CORRECT (OR NOT APPLICABLE)
- HOW THE SPECIMEN IS LABELLED (INCLUDING PATIENT NAME)
- WHETHER THERE ARE ANY EQUIPMENT PROBLEMS TO BE ADDRESSED
- SURGEON, ANAESTHESIA PROFESSIONAL AND NURSE REVIEW THE KEY CONCERNS FOR RECOVERY AND MANAGEMENT OF THIS PATIENT

'How does it work?'

The checklist separates every operation into three categories; the 'sign in', 'time out' and 'sign out'. A single person, usually the theatre nurse, is responsible for running through the list, however, any healthcare worker participating in the operation can be responsible. During each phase, the checklist coordinator must be allowed to perform the WHO checks. Over time, as teams work together these checks can be verbalised without conscious interruptions such that the checklist is incorporated into every procedure, with minimal disruption and optimal work efficiency.

'What is involved at "Sign in"?'

'Sign In' takes place in the period before the induction of anaesthesia. It usually involves the anaesthetist and nursing staff, at the very least. The following checks are made:

Before induction of anaesthesia ▶▶▶▶▶▶▶▶▶

SIGN IN

☐ PATIENT HAS CONFIRMED
  • IDENTITY
  • SITE
  • PROCEDURE
  • CONSENT

☐ SITE MARKED/NOT APPLICABLE

☐ ANAESTHESIA SAFETY CHECK COMPLETED

☐ PULSE OXIMETER ON PATIENT AND FUNCTIONING

DOES PATIENT HAVE A:

KNOWN ALLERGY?
☐ NO
☐ YES

DIFFICULT AIRWAY/ASPIRATION RISK?
☐ NO
☐ YES, AND EQUIPMENT/ASSISTANCE AVAILABLE

RISK OF >500ML BLOOD LOSS
(7ML/KG IN CHILDREN)?
☐ NO
☐ YES, AND ADEQUATE INTRAVENOUS ACCESS
   AND FLUIDS PLANNED

1. **Patient has confirmed identity, site, procedure and consent**: These are verbally confirmed with checks made against hospital number and signed consent forms. This ensures the correct procedure at the correct site is performed on the correct patient. The box is left unchecked in the case of emergencies if a patient is incapacitated and no close family/friends are available;

2. **Site marked**: The site should be marked by the operating surgeon with a permanent marker and is confirmed during the checklist;

3. **Anaesthesia safety check**: The anaesthesia check confirms with the anaesthetic staff that an anaesthesia safety check has been completed. This typically involves the ABCDE's: Airway equipment, Breathing system (including oxygen and inhalational

agents), suCtion, Drugs and devices and Emergency medications, equipment and assistance in order to confirm their availability and functioning;

4. **Pulse oximeter**: The presence of a correctly placed and working pulse oximeter is checked. It should be visible to all staff and, where available, have an audible alarm system present to alert the staff to the patient's pulse and oxygen saturation;

5. **Allergy**: This is asked directly to the anaesthetic staff to ensure they have made the necessary checks themselves; and

6. **Difficult airway**: This is asked directly to the anaesthetic staff who may use any number of airway checks such as the Mallampati score, thyromental distance or Bellhouse-Doré score. The risk of aspiration must also be evaluated.

Risk of >500 mL blood loss: If there is ≥500 mL blood loss, or equivalent in children, it is recommended that at least two large-bore IV cannulas be present (or a central venous catheter). Appropriate fluids or blood must also be confirmed and available for resuscitation if required. The estimated blood loss is also reviewed during the 'Time Out' check.

'What is involved at "Time Out"?'

Time out is the period after induction and before the surgical incision (Time Out). This involves the following checks:

Before skin incision ▶▶▶▶▶▶▶▶▶▶▶▶▶▶

TIME OUT

☐ CONFIRM ALL TEAM MEMBERS HAVE INTRODUCED THEMSELVES BY NAME AND ROLE

☐ SURGEON, ANAESTHESIA PROFESSIONAL AND NURSE VERBALLY CONFIRM
- PATIENT
- SITE
- PROCEDURE

ANTICIPATED CRITICAL EVENTS

☐ SURGEON REVIEWS: WHAT ARE THE CRITICAL OR UNEXPECTED STEPS, OPERATIVE DURATION, ANTICIPATED BLOOD LOSS?

☐ ANAESTHESIA TEAM REVIEWS: ARE THERE ANY PATIENT-SPECIFIC CONCERNS?

☐ NURSING TEAM REVIEWS: HAS STERILITY (INCLUDING INDICATOR RESULTS) BEEN CONFIRMED? ARE THERE EQUIPMENT ISSUES OR ANY CONCERNS?

HAS ANTIBIOTIC PROPHYLAXIS BEEN GIVEN WITHIN THE LAST 60 MINUTES?
☐ YES
☐ NOT APPLICABLE

IS ESSENTIAL IMAGING DISPLAYED?
☐ YES
☐ NOT APPLICABLE

1. **Confirm all team members have introduced themselves by name and role**: Given the frequent rotation of team members (team members turnover is rapid) and shifts demanding on-calls and night shifts this is an important step. The introduction also applies to students and any other personnel who may join an operation or the theatre list at any point.

2. **Surgeon, anaesthetist and nurse verbally confirm: Patient, site and procedure**: This is typically known as the 'surgical pause'. Prior to the operation starting the checklist (perform checklist before the operation begins) coordinator will verbally confirm the patient's name, procedure, site and patient position.

3. **Anticipated critical events**: An important and efficient discussion takes place between the surgical, anaesthetic and nursing staff regarding any anticipated dangers, operative plans and equipment issues.

4. **Antibiotic prophylaxis**: There is strong and accepted evidence that antibiotic prophylaxis for wound infection is most effective within 1 hour before the incision. The checklist coordinator should therefore control this specifically, and if antibiotics have not been given, they should be administered before the incision takes place. If >60 mins have occurred, redosing should be considered. The N/A box is checked if antibiotics are not indicated.

Essential imaging: Imaging is particularly important in orthopaedic, tumour and spinal procedures amongst others. Imaging requirements should be checked with the surgeon and, if needed, confirmed that they are present and visible in the room.

'What is involved at "Sign Out"?'

The 'Sign Out' is the period during or immediately after wound closure – but before removing the patient from the operating room – and represents a debrief of the procedure. This involves the following checks:

Before patient leaves operating room

SIGN OUT

NURSE VERBALLY CONFIRMS WITH THE TEAM:

☐ THE NAME OF THE PROCEDURE RECORDED

☐ THAT INSTRUMENT, SPONGE AND NEEDLE COUNTS ARE CORRECT (OR NOT APPLICABLE)

☐ HOW THE SPECIMEN IS LABELLED (INCLUDING PATIENT NAME)

☐ WHETHER THERE ARE ANY EQUIPMENT PROBLEMS TO BE ADDRESSED

☐ SURGEON, ANAESTHESIA PROFESSIONAL AND NURSE REVIEW THE KEY CONCERNS FOR RECOVERY AND MANAGEMENT OF THIS PATIENT

1. **The name of the procedure recorded:** Since procedures may change, or be expanded upon, the checklist coordinator should confirm the exact procedure(s) performed;

2. **Instrument, sponge and needle counts are correct**: This is typically performed nearing the end of the operative procedure, usually by the scrub nurse. If the count is not satisfactory, the team should be alerted to allow for appropriate measures to take place such as checking the drapes, waste and wound;

3. **Specimen labelling**: Incorrect sample labelling is a common and disastrous outcome for a patient, who is likely to have been through a trialling procedure and/ or experience. The patient's name, specimen description and site markings should therefore be checked verbally;

4. **Equipment problems**: Identifying failing or faulty equipment, including instruments, allows recycling of these to prevent further use in future procedures; and

5. **Review of concerns for recovery and management**: The surgical, anaesthetic and nursing teams review the postoperative management plans, particularly any operative or anaesthetic concerns that may impact upon the patient. This ensures effective communication and anticipation of events that may affect the patient.

4. INTRODUCTION TO THE PORTFOLIO STATION

The surgical portfolio now represents an essential requirement and is a vital part of the core surgical training application process. The portfolio should be a reflection of the candidates' achievements in surgical training, clinical practice and continuing professional development. Although a daunting and exhaustive preparation process, you should view the portfolio station as an opportunity to demonstrate with full conviction why you deserve to be a surgical trainee. This is the station that you have the most opportunity to identify potential weaknesses and address them. It is also the station for which you can carry out the greatest preparations in order to make your application as strong as possible. The scoring proportion of this station mirrors that of the clinical and management stations, constituting 33% of the final result. The portfolio assessment is based upon three avenues of assessment:

1. The application form as a formative assessment of your achievements for which you must show evidence;
2. The physical portfolio itself and its contents; and
3. The answers to the portfolio station interview.

After registering at the interview venue, your portfolio will be taken shortly before the interview is set to take place. The interviewers in the portfolio station then have the daunting task of working through the relevant contents of your portfolio. They will, where possible, mark areas on an assessment sheet before you are called in, as well as prepare questions depending on the contents of your portfolio.

> *The portfolio station was the station I enjoyed the most. The interviewers helped me stay calm and relaxed as it was my first station of the day. I had spent hours and hours constantly flicking through every section of the portfolio ensuring not only that I knew every page within it, but also preparing for the potential questions that might arise. It is the station that consumed a lot of my time in preparation; not only do you have to provide evidence for every aspect of your surgical training but also ensure it is in the most organised and user-friendly format for the interviewers.*

4.1 EXAMPLE PORTFOLIO STRUCTURE I

Trying to make sense of how to structure your portfolio – that neatly categorizes your relevant documents and achievements in a well-organised and well-presented manner – can be a difficult and frustrating task. Remember, this is your extended surgical CV, therefore ensure your strengths are adequately sectioned and highlighted. As you organise your portfolio, clear weaknesses will become apparent allowing you an opportunity to either address these and fill gaps in the portfolio, or prepare answers for the questions that may arise. The following is an example structure to help you make a start in organising your portfolio.

The deanery will make clear to you how they would like you to organize your portfolio. Do not deviate from this in anyway, make it easy for the examiner to find all the relevant information in the manner that they have asked.

Next is an example from the past of portfolio structures to give you an idea; however, always refer to the deanery website to obtain the most up-to-date version of arranging your portfolio. They will also include a marking scheme to give you an idea of what scores higher and what is acceptable (see also Portfolio structure II: Summaries).

Formal Documents

1. CV
2. GMC certificate
3. FACD 5.1 (FY1 competencies)
4. Passport copies and photographs
5. Medical degree certificate and diploma supplement
6. BSc/Postgraduate certificates (If appropriate)
7. MRCS examinations A/B (If appropriate)

Prizes

1. Research, e.g., poster, presentations, etc.
2. Academic, e.g., examinations, essays, etc.
3. Extracurricular, e.g., elective, sporting honours, etc.

Research and Audit*

1. Publications (Printed article in published pdf format)
2. Oral Presentations (Colour powerpoint handouts)
3. Posters (1 Page A4 summary)
4. Audit (Colour powerpoint handouts)

Courses

1. Immediate Life Support
2. Advanced Life Support
3. Advanced Trauma Life Support
4. Basic Surgical Skills Course
5. Care of the Critically Ill Surgical Patient

Leadership and Management

1. Doctors Mess President
2. Foundation School (FY1/FY2) representative
3. Involvement in rota organisation
4. Leadership courses
5. Mentoring courses and mentor groups
6. Team leader for sports teams

Eportfolio and eLogbook

- Eportfolio contents page — Core procedures summary (include best first)
- DOPS Summary (include best first) — Mini CEX Summary (include best first)
- Case Based Discussion Summary (include best first) — TAB assessments
- Developing the Clinical Teacher Assessment (place in the teaching section also)
- Clinical Leadership Development
  1. Reflective practice
  2. Clinical Supervisor Reports
  3. Educational/Academic Reports
- eLogbook (Assisted and performed procedures)

Teaching and feedback

1. Teach the teacher
2. Train the trainer
3. Informal teaching sessions (dates of teaching, titles, audience type, number of attendants)
4. Formal teaching sessions (dates of teaching, titles, audience type, number of attendants)
5. Feedback forms
6. Teaching assessments from eportfolio

Extracurricular

1. Sporting interests
2. Musical involement
3. Debating
4. Religious involement
5. Humanitarian efforts

References

Application references

Character references

Formal Documents

1. CV
2. GMC certificate
3. FACD 5.1 (FY1 competencies)
4. Passport copies and photographs

5. Medical degree certificate and diploma supplement
6. BSc/Postgraduate certificates (if appropriate)
7. MRCS Examinations A/B (if appropriate)

The formal documents section should house your professional qualifications, for which you should keep at least two copies of each within the portfolio. These documents should include but not be limited to:

CV

A succinct and well presented CV that allows the interviewers to quickly scan through your achievements to date. Keep several copies of this so that all the interviewers (usually 2) can read through at their leisure.

GMC Certificate

Ensure that original copies of the provisional and full registration GMC certificates are present with multiple copies. This will be more for the administration aspect of the interview, but demonstrates a well-organised portfolio that makes all relevant documents available.

FACD 5.1 (FY1 competencies)

Ensure that original copies of the FACD 5.1 document are present with multiple copies. This has in the past been used to cross check your NHS portfolio, and is not just for administration purposes.

Medical Degree Certificate with Diploma Supplement

Your formal qualification certificate, along with copies, should be available along with the diploma supplement. This outlines the various marks and modules that make up your finals qualification and should be present alongside the degree certificate itself.

BSc/Postgraduate Degrees

If you have completed a BSc, or any other degree qualification, this should also be made available. Remember to include the certificate and the degree supplement that outlines a break down of marks in your first class, 2:1, etc.

MRCS Examinations

If you have completed any part of the MRCS examination, include this also in your formal documents section. The certificate can take long to arrive, therefore your formal results letter is also acceptable.

Prizes

1. Research, e.g., poster, presentations, etc.
2. Academic, e.g., examinations, essays, etc.
3. Extracurricular, e.g., elective, sporting honours, debates, etc.

It is always impressive to begin your portfolio with a listing of any prizes that you have achieved, with a brief explanation of what the prize was for and the competitive nature of the award. National prizes score highly with honours, distinctions, merits also being variously awarded. Place the original and photocopies of the prize certificates. If you were awarded something other than a certificate, such as a plaque, cup, and so forth, it is not unreasonable to bring this with you but it may be more manageable to include a photo in place of the physical item.

Research and Audit/QI*

1. Publications (printed article in published pdf format)
2. Oral Presentations (colour powerpoint handouts)
3. Posters (1 page A4 summary)
4. Audit (colour powerpoint handouts)

Increasingly important is a demonstration of formal research and audit projects that you have conducted. For candidates that have invested time in original research, or have successfully published peer-reviewed journal articles, this is a show of strength and credibility to your application. Include the formal published copy of your article (front page only with authorship) and ensure you are completely familiar with the research questions, methodology, statistics and conclusions. Presentations can be shortened into handouts with several slides per page (ideally single page that includes an opening slide with your name), whilst posters can also be reduced to 1-page summaries. Do not print reams of all your papers, posters and presentations, as you will be penalized for this.

For candidates that do not have any formal research, do not panic! Remember there is still time to contribute to this section if you have identified it as an area of weakness, and perhaps more importantly, it should be a question that you should prepare to be challenged upon. For each article of research, presentation or poster include the following information: Your involvement in conceiving the research idea, data collection, contribution to writing the paper and presentation of findings.

*Audit/QI

Also of increasing importance are audits and quality improvement projects, particularly those that have closed the loop and made an impact upon clinical practice. The audit presentation, with a short summary, should be included as well as details as to where the audit has been presented. For each audit include a statement such as:

> *I conceived the audit idea, organised and performed the data collection, data analysis, implementation of change to current practice and presentation of this audit at a clinical governance meeting. I have closed the audit cycle loop and improved the quality of consent forms in accordance with the British Association of Orthopaedic guidelines.*

Courses

1. Immediate Life Support
2. Advanced Life Support
3. Advanced Trauma Life Support
4. Basic Surgical Skills Course
5. Care of the Critically Ill Surgical Patient

The courses subsection demonstrates your commitment to surgery and is worth including early in your portfolio. Virtually all candidates will be aware of the minimum courses that need to be completed and therefore it is now almost essential that you try to complete the 'Basic Surgical Skills Course', 'Advanced Trauma Life Support' and the 'Advanced Life Support' courses well before your interview. The certificates for these can take several months to arrive, although placing the letter of participation that you receive on the day of these courses is just as valid as the formal certificate itself. There also other courses that will contribute to your application such as the 'Care of the Critically ill Surgical Patient', although they can be difficult to enroll in for juniors, which is understood by the interviewers. If you have a clear idea of the surgical career you wish to undertake, the Royal College of Surgeons has regular listings for career-specific courses though again these are not by any means mandatory, and often premature if taken at a foundation level of training. Foundation level courses in surgery that may be relevant also include:

- Basic Surgical Skills
- START Surgery
- ATLS, Surgical Skills for Surgeons
- RCS Summer School in Anatomy
- Practical Skills for Medical Students
- So you want to be an Orthopaedic Surgeon
- Clinical Skills for Examining Orthopaedic Patients or Equivalent surgically orientated courses
- Temporal bone course
- FESS (Sinus surgery) course
- Head and Neck anatomy/surgical dissection course
- Urology Courses: National Catheter Education Programme (NCEP)

Eportfolio and eLogbook

- Eportfolio contents page — Core procedures summary (include best first)
- DOPS Summary (include best first) — Mini CEX Summary (include best first)
- Case Based Discussion Summary (include best first) — TAB assessments
- Developing the Clinical Teacher Assessment (Place a copy of this in the teaching section also)
- Clinical Leadership Development
  1. Reflective practice
  2. Clinical Supervisor Reports
  3. Educational/Academic Reports
- eLogbook (Assisted and performed procedures)

The NHS eportfolio section should be treated as a miniportfolio in its own right. Ensure that this section is highly organised, with a clear contents section that allows the interviewer to quickly move to the appropriate section of assessments. Your Work based assessments should be divided based on type such as mini-CEX, CBDs, and so forth. Include the best at the very front since interviewers will not have time to review more than 1-2 of each of these, however, they will note the scores and feedback for those assessments that they do review.

All candidates should have a printout and signed logbook of surgical procedures that they have assisted in. Ensure that you have an eLogbook and ISCP account (the ISCP account is more relevant when you become a core surgical trainee, however, having an account shows you are abreast of how surgical training is conducted). Core Surgical Training has reached such a level of competition that interviewers will now even take note of operations that you have performed, rather than just assisted in.

Leadership and Management

  1. Doctors Mess President
  2. Foundation School (FY1/FY2) representative
  3. Involvement in rota organisation
  4. Leadership courses

5. Mentoring courses and mentor groups

6. Team leader for sports teams

The leadership and management section can be a difficult section to complete depending on your activities within and outside of the hospital. There are specific courses such as the mentoring and leadership courses that are directly relevant in this section. Other activities, such as being the lead for medical student teaching, is also a relevant activity that demonstrates your teaching and leadership qualities. This is also a popular area of questioning that will investigate how you employ your attributes of leadership.

Teaching and feedback

1. Teach the teacher

2. Train the trainer

3. Informal teaching sessions (dates of teaching, titles, audience type, number of attendants)

4. Formal teaching sessions (dates of teaching, titles, audience type, number of attendants)

5. Feedback forms

6. Teaching assessments from eportfolio

The most overlooked section of the portfolio by candidates is the teaching and feedback aspect. This section should include any informal, and most importantly, formal teaching that you have organised. Informal teaching includes any inpromptu teaching, such as bedside finals teaching for medical students. A formal teaching programme would be scheduled, regularly timetabled sessions for a set audience. Teaching materials used should be included along with teaching timetables, lesson plans and most importantly formal feedback from your audience. These should include the title of your session, date, time and clear areas for feedback, including free text boxes.

Extracurricular

1. Sporting interests

2. Musical involement

3. Debating

4. Religious involement

5. Humanitarian efforts

Well-rounded candidates, who are able to link their extracurricular activities to furthering their surgical attributes, perform exceeding well at interview when they include these in their portfolio. Relevant achievements outside of medicine should be included in this section, with appropriate evidence.

References

Application references

Character references

Lastly, written formal references are required by the administrative office and copies of these should be available. However, you should also include character references with previous surgical consultants – this is an additional support to your application that not many other candidates will think to include.

4.2 EXAMPLE PORTFOLIO STRUCTURE II: SUMMARIES

Summarising your portfolio to ensure that it is easy for the examiners to find the evidence of your achievements is key. Candidates regularly print off entire paper articles, full lengths of presentations and posters. This padding out of the portfolio will always be detrimental to your score. The following are some examples summaries that can be placed in each section – again strictly follow the guidance of the deanery website, which will always make clear exactly how they would like you to arrange your portfolio order.

Publications, Oral presentations and posters

Publications

1. It doesn't 'come with the job': violence against doctors at work must stop
   SSDubb
   BMJ 2015; 350 doi: http://dx.doi.org/10.1136/bmj.h2780
2. The Marconi Sign: The Value of Clinical Examination
   SS Dubb, list other authors as appropriate
   British Medical Journal 2012 Aug
   www.bmj.com/content/339/bmj.b5448/rr/597208

Oral Presentations

1. Aspirin desensitisation: Our Experience
   SSDubb list other authors as appropriate
   Scottish Otolaryngological Society ENT Meeting, Dublane, May 2015
2. Blood Pressure and Renal Cytokines Improve After Bariatrics Surgery
   SSDubb, list other authors as appropriate
   British Renal Society Annual Conference Manchester 2010

Posters

1. CT Scan Consideration for Occult Skull Fracture in Paediatric Head Trauma
   SSDubb, list other authors as appropriate
   JTG London 2019 **(Prize Winner)**
2. Impact of accurate clinical in Oral and Maxillofacial surgery
   SSDubb, list other authors as appropriate
   JTG London 2018

Audit and quality improvement projects

Closed loop audit

Audit of CBCT referrals for exodontia compared to European Commission Guidelines

Dubb SS et al

Name of Hospital Trust

Audit Loop: CLOSED **Presentation:** Regional Meeting

Audit standard: European Commission Guidelines

Impact on clinical practice: Improved understanding of CBCT indications for exodontia, cost reduction and training within department.

Open loop audit

Appropriate Use of Intravenous Fluids in Surgical Patients Based on NICE Guidelines

Dubb SS et al

Name of Hospital Trust

Audit Loop: 1st cycle **Presentation:** Regional Meeting

Audit standard: NICE guidelines

Impact on clinical practice: Improved the quality and safety of fluid prescription according to Royal College of Physician Guidelines

Quality improvement project

Ward Round: Plan, Do, Study, Act Cycle of Ward Round Notes

Audit Loop: 1st loop complete **Presentation:** Regional Meeting

Dubb SS et al

Name of Hospital Trust

Audit Loop: CLOSED **Presentation:** Regional Meeting

Audit standard: NICE guidelines

Impact on clinical practice: Improved the quality and safety ward round notes according to Royal College of Physician Guidelines

Audit summary page

The following is an example of summarising your audit

Audit title: an audit of adherence to a modified ward round checklist based on Royal College of Physicians' ward rounds in medicine principles for best practice

AUDIT LOOP: CLOSED   **PRESENTATION:** Regional governance meeting

LEAD: Sukhpreet S Dubb   **SUPERVISOR:** As appropriate

LOCATION: As appropriate

REASON: Ensure that an efficient and safe ward round was being conducted by rotating senior and junior members of the surgical team

DESCRIPTION AND INVOLVEMENT: Conceived, organised, performed data collection, performed analysis, conducted implementation and presentation of this audit at regional clinical governance meeting.

AUDIT STANDARD: Royal College of Physicians Ward rounds in medicine Principles for best practice

DATA COLLECTION: 90 patients between Apr–Aug 2019

INCLUSION CRITERIA: All paediatric surgery inpatients seen on ward round

EXCLUSION CRITERIA: None–paediatric surgery patients on ward round

TIME PERIOD: Apr–Aug 2019

1st CYCLE RESULTS: Fluid balance status and nutrition (80%), drug chart review (70%), team introductions performed in 44%, Ward round pre-preparation in 40%, jobs/actions assigned in 24%

2nd CYCLE RESULTS: Fluid balance status and nutrition (100%), drug chart review (95%), team introductions performed in 80%, Ward round pre-preparation in 100%, jobs/actions assigned in 90%

INTERVENTION: Placement of audit and results in patient rooms as well as Doctors' offices. New portable ward round check-list to be placed in jobs book.

IMPACT ON CLINICAL PRACTICE:

Change in department guidelines for ward round check lists:

- New modified ward round check list a permanent fixture
- Part of induction of new team members
- Regular audit cycle for junior doctors

Teaching summary examples

1. **Oral and Maxillofacial Teaching Co-ordinator (Date)**
   Name of hospital trust

2. **Plastic Surgery Teaching Co-ordinator (Date)**
   Aberdeen Royal Infirmary

3. **Specialist Study Module in Surgery: Medical Student supervisor (Date)**
   (Name of medical school)

4. **Surgery Clinical Teaching Fellow (Date)**
   Formal 9 Week Undergraduate Surgical Teaching Curriculum to Undergraduate Medical Students
   (Name of medical school)

5. Undergraduate Finals Teaching **(Date)**
   (Name of medical school)

6. Year 3 Mock OSCE Examination and Teaching **(Date)**
   (Name of medical school)

7. Year 3 OSCE Tutoring **(Date)**
   (Name of medical school)

8. Preclinical Teaching Tutorials **(Date)**
   (Name of medical school)

9. Hockey Coaching for Under 13's **(Date)**
   Name of club

Training posts example	Dates
FY2 in Accident & Emergency	Feb–Aug 2020
Name of hospital	
FY2 in General Practice	Nov–Feb 2019
Name of hospital	
FY2 in Trauma and Orthopaedics	Aug–Nov 2019
Newham General Hospital	
FY1 in GI Surgery	Apr–Aug 2018
Name of hospital	
FY1 in Breast Surgery	Dec–Apr 2018
Name of hospital	
FY1 in General Medicine	Aug–Dec 2018
Name of hospital	

4.3 AUDIT

'What is a clinical audit?'

A clinical audit compares a current given clinical practice against a given gold standard and validates how closely we are performing guidelines. It is a way to systematically review clinical practice, identify areas of deficiency and intervene to allow standards to be maintained in clinical care. It forms one of the pillars of clinical governance.

'What is the difference between a clinical audit and clinical research?'

The aim of a clinical audit is comparison of current clinical practice to a recognised, set gold standard. Clinical research aims to answer or disprove a question (null hypothesis) with the aim of establishing or contributing to best practice. Research produces new knowledge or affirms existing results whilst a clinical audit aims to improve practice. It is specific to a particular area of clinical practice and results are not transferrable across other settings. Clinical audit is also an on-going process with continual review and comparison, whilst research is usually a singular process with larger or more advanced studies exploring other avenues. Clinical research itself can be audited to ensure high quality work is being implemented.

'What are the gold standards used in clinical audit?'

The gold standards used to compare clinical practice are usually national standards that have been formulated by a clinical institution or authoritative body. This may include the National Institute for Clinical Excellence (NICE), British Orthopaedics Association (BOA), Scottish Intercollegiate Guidelines Network (SIGN) or the Royal College of Surgeons. An example would be the guidelines from the Royal College of Surgeons that outline the minimum information that should be recorded on operating records. This is a gold standard guideline to which every surgeon should adhere to.

'What is the difference between an audit and a survey?'

A survey primarily collects data for a given clinical practice or service, the information may then be analysed and used to implement changes where necessary. There is, however, no comparison to a recognised gold standard or guideline.

'What is an audit cycle?'

An audit begins with the identification of an area of clinical practice that may be suboptimal. A corresponding gold standard is then identified which can be used to compare the standard of clinical practice. Data is then collated and the results analysed to identify excellence and deficiency. Interventions are formulated and facilitated to rectify areas that are not adhering to the gold standard. A re-audit then takes place, following a reasonable period of adjustment, to review the level of improvement of clinical practice and how closely it resembles the set guidelines. This is often termed 'closing the loop'. This describes a continuing process that should be repeated in a cyclical manner in order to ensure the highest standards of clinical practice.

'Why is clinical audit important?'

The main outcome of a clinical audit is to ensure the highest standards are being maintained in clinical practice, and that service provision is therefore of the highest quality. This can be difficult to know or prove without the use of a clinical audit which allows areas of weakness to be identified, and provides recognised information that demonstrates the effectiveness of the given service. Other benefits include improving service delivery even further through education, training and improved, more efficient resource management.

'What are the area of clinical practice that can be audited?'

The breadth of clinical practice that can undergo audit is limitless and often subjective depending on what areas of service may appear to be deficient. There are, however, three broad areas under which an audit can be classified.

- The structure: Resources and personnel organisation
- The process: The utilisation of a service's resources
- The outcome: The impact the service has on the end user, usually the patient receiving a treatment

Background information

The stages of a clinical audit are summarised next:

- Identify an area of practice that may be substandard
- Identify a relevant guideline, or gold standard, suitable for comparison
- Design a collection proforma that allows data collection in a comparable format with a given time frame for data collection
- Undertake data collection
- Compare the data to the gold standard
- Identify areas that are substandard and why they may be so. Formulate interventions to improve these areas
- Implement changes through various channels
- Re-audit after a reasonable period to allow changes to take place, and review the standard of service and how close it may be to the gold standard

Clinical audit projects are more successful if they involve as many members of the service providers as possible, this ranges from the clinical staff, non-clinical management, service users, audit office, and so on. By involving as many different categories of personnel in the audit work, you increase the chance of uptake and implementation of changes to better the service as a whole.

4.4 COMMITMENT TO SURGERY

A career in surgery is demanding, exhausting, challenging but ultimately rewarding. The training period can take anywhere between 8–12 years after foundation training with many levels of application, appraisal and examination. The competition for places is fierce at every level and the core surgical training application is the first formal step onto the surgical career pathway. Part of the portfolio station interview questions will challenge your commitment to surgery and whether you have fully considered the implications and sacrifice required. Being able to give genuine and well-constructed answers, using your portfolio to supplement and support your application, is the key to setting yourself apart from all other candidates.

'Why do you want to be a surgeon?'

The field of surgery entices me at a clinical, practical and managerial level. Clinically, I find an equal fascination between medicine and surgery in acquiring the knowledge that underlies disease, and using this to make accurate diagnoses. However, I was frustrated by the increasing dependence upon outside factors such as the efficacy and pharmacology of the drugs used to treat a patient in whom I had successfully diagnosed pneumonia. In contrast to this, I was strongly attracted by correctly diagnosing a patient with a hernia, practising specific parts of an operation, such as knot tying, and then being able to employ this in the theatre to directly manage a patient's pathology. Patients are also understandably anxious about any operative procedure and therefore demand the very best in communication skills to tackle their concerns and expectations, which is a great attraction for me. The nature of surgery is direct, with visible action that benefits patients almost immediately after intervention.

The practical aspects of surgery also present a unique physical challenge that requires the simultaneous memorisation of surgical steps involved in an operation, as well as the different surgical techniques needed to complete these steps. Surgery also involves various technologies and research, which is an exciting prospect that aids the diagnosis and intervention of patients with surgical disease. I particularly enjoy practising and honing a surgical skill so that at the time of the operation, I can successfully execute this particular task at the appropriate time.

Finally, there is an important management side of surgery that demands self-discipline and organisation. Successful surgeons are able to be operative not only independently, but also as part of a team – not just in the operating theatre but also as part of a multidisciplinary team drawing on the respective expertise of other specialties to treat a patient.

'What do you least like about surgery?'

Although I am firmly committed to pursuing a career in surgery, I am realistic about the other challenges that I would face in training. Surgery involves a long and arduous training pathway requiring commitment and persistence. I have been somewhat concerned about potential training issues when speaking to my peers already in core surgical training. All surgical trainees face potential surgical exposure issues, given the restriction of EWTD. However, I have changed my focus to obtaining quality training rather than just quantity in numbers, which should help to tackle this issue. Following medical school, it has been a welcome break to be away from examinations and revisions, however, there are a number of challenging examinations that must be successfully passed in order to progress along this specialty. Even after examinations, surgery truly involves lifelong learning; even after mastering examinations and surgical procedures, there is always room for improvement in efficiency and economy of movement. As surgical technology and research advances, new techniques and methodologies become apparent requiring investment in these new procedures.

I am also aware of the on-call commitments in surgery that will continue up to and after completion of training. This will include long day shifts, weekends on-call and night shifts. As time has progressed, I have become more adapted to this working lifestyle, however, as my commitments and priorities change, I am aware of the impact this is likely to have on my family and social life, especially when balancing commitments such as marriage and children. I have also noticed that patient expectations can far exceed the capabilities of modern surgery, and this requires a truthful and realistic discussion which patients are always ready for.

'Demonstrate your interest in surgery'

From a clinical perspective, I have completed a 4 month in breast surgery, colorectal surgery and trauma and orthopaedics providing me with one year of surgical training. This involved general surgery on-call and night shifts, affording me an excellent exposure to the breadth and depth of surgery. Within this period, I have successfully logged more than 100 surgical procedures as an assistant, with a small number of operations in which I was the primary surgeon. This was despite working at a busy teaching hospital with considerable clinical commitments on the ward. During my elective, I also worked at a trauma centre in South Africa and in the United States, giving me excellent hands-on technical experience in two very different, yet renowned, health centres in the world.

Academically, I have invested my spare time in a research project at the local surgical unit from which I have been able to publish a peer-reviewed research paper. During medical school, I also undertook a BSc in surgery, completing a surgical project which led to an abstract and poster presentation.

I have also successfully completed two surgical audits looking at operation notes and consent forms in surgery. For both of these audits, I closed the loop of the audit and was able to positively impact clinical practice. I am currently presenting these audits as a poster presentation at a local research conference. Finally, I have booked and am currently revising for the MRCS examination part A. As part of my continuing personal professional development, I have successfully completed a basic surgical skills course and an Advanced Trauma Life Support course. The basic surgical skills course also involved a microsurgery taster session, which I found very interesting and has sparked an interest in a potential career in plastic surgery.

Finally, I have developed my interest in surgical education by setting up a formal teaching programme for the medical students on rotation at my hospital. I liased with the teaching coordinator of the hospital and was able to organise regular scheduled teachings for the 3rd clinical students that involved lectures and bedside clinical teaching. I was given excellent feedback for this from the students, and was lucky enough to receive a teaching award from the hospital based on the teaching feedback. I am a strong advocate of e-learning and have completed several surgery modules on e-learning for health and doctors.net websites part of my developing surgical education.

'Where do you see yourself in 10 years' time in this specialty?'

After 10 years of surgical training, I would hope to be a senior surgical registrar close to obtaining my certificate of completion of training. My aim is to obtain a position in a tertiary teaching hospital which would allow me to interact with a diverse mix of patients and presentations. I would also relish the challenges of a busy surgical department requiring a strong leadership position, delegation to teams involving junior registrars, core surgical trainees, senior house officers and foundation year trainees. I have an interest in plastic surgery and in 10 years' time this would be an opportune moment to consider fellowships in craniofacial surgery and facial defects. I have researched several of these programmes in Australia as well as received excellent feedback from senior trainees. I have an interest in surgical education and would therefore be very keen to be involved in delivering a regular teaching programme to medical students and even junior trainees.

'What has influenced your deanery choices?'

In making my deanery choices, I have looked at a number of factors to aid my final decision between deaneries, although I would be delighted to work anywhere as a core surgical trainee. The experience of past surgical trainees is important to me as a rough guide to which deaneries house the best surgical trainers and active teachers in surgery. I wish to attend a deanery which caters to a large and diverse population mix, so that I may see a large and varied number of surgical presentations. I would also hope to have access to teaching hospitals that have research interests so that I may expand upon the research work that I have already started.

From an academic perspective, the teaching programme offered by the deanery is also very important as I know this can be very varied. I would hope to join a deanery that has a regular and up-to-date teaching programme with a variation in anatomy, surgical theory and practical skill development. I am also very interested in being involved with a local medical school to further develop my interest in surgical education.

As part of my continuing professional development, the demands of the deanery – such as work-based assessments and successful ARCP reviews – has also helped to guide my decision. The number of courses that the deanery offers, such as simulation-based teaching, leadership, teaching and e-learning courses is also very important.

4.5 CRITICAL APPRAISAL

It is now becoming much more uncommon for candidates to be asked to perform a critical appraisal of a paper. The process does not fit into the current format of interview stations, and candidates wouldn't have time to read through a paper and perform a reasonable critique, which itself would prevent other questions from being asked. Some deaneries have in the past given short reports or reviews, although even these have been scarce in the past few interview cycles. However, it is not unreasonable to ask candidates their method of critiquing a paper. Indeed, the very best candidates – who have evidence of publications in their portfolio – have been asked how they would perform a critical appraisal of their own work. Critical appraisal does not simply run through the skeletal framework of a paper and review the introduction, methodology, discussions and so forth. There are much more important fundamental questions that need to be reviewed first, and this creates the distinction between candidates who actually understand how to critically review scientific work from those who have a rudimentary understanding. We have therefore included a run through of how to perform the critical appraisal of a paper.

'Is the research question relevant?'

The research study must be based around an important topic which contributes something significant to the subject matter. This is entirely subjective and for the reader to decide whether the question being investigated is of interest.

'Does the study contribute anything new?'

The majority of scientific work is based upon previous studies, with new ideas and knowledge being derived from predecessors' work. This is not by any means to suggest such work is not helpful, indeed incremental advances and validation of previous work is carried out in this way, which can expand the original study's clinical context or target population.

'What type of research question does the study pose?'

The most important focus of a critical appraisal is determining how well the study addresses the research question that has been posed. It is therefore fundamental that you identify what this is, and then compare how well the study has been designed to answer this, as well as the importance and relevance of their findings. Each research question should have three facets to it, including:

1. Population of patients to be studied;
2. The intervention; and
3. The outcome of interest.

Was the study designed appropriately for the research question?

The hierarchy of the study design is important here, and there is a well-established order that includes meta-analysis and randomised control trials at the top, and anecdotal evidence at the bottom. However, not every research study can perform a randomised control trial for the research question being posed, and indeed, it may not always be appropriate. For this situation, other study designs need to be chosen, such as observational studies that are more appropriate when answering how frequently a disease occurs, or case control studies that are more appropriate for very rare diseases, and so forth.

'Was bias adequately controlled?'

The effect of bias on a study can either affect the precision of the study results (most often random error), or cause an over/under estimation of the final conclusion (systematic error). It is therefore important to reduce random and systematic bias as much as possible through meticulous conduct of the study, data collection and results analysis.

'Did the study adhere to an original protocol?'

Studies that build upon previous work should aim to replicate the work so that reproducible results can be compared across other work. Deviating from the original protocol will affect the validity of such results. The most common reasons for such deviations to occur include:

1. Failing to recruit enough participants for a study;
2. Changes to the inclusion and exclusion criteria;
3. Differences in the interventions provided; and
4. Follow-up differences.

'Was the statistical analysis conducted appropriately?'

Although not always easy to assess, the rationale for why a statistical analysis was performed should be included in the methodology section of a paper. An important principle to check in a paper is whether an 'intention to treat' approach was used or 'as per protocol' analysis was adopted. Ideally, patients should be analysed based on the group they were allocated to, regardless of whether they received the intervention or not. If participants were non-compliant, then the study can be limited to those participants to those who adhered to the study protocol. The disadvantage of this latter analysis is a high risk of selection bias.

'Do the conclusions match the results?'

It can be very tempting, as the author of a study, to emphasise or downplay a significant finding in order to support a given conclusion in the discussion section of a paper. They may also make unreasonable assumptions, or apply their results out of context. A close review of the results, both significant and not significant, is therefore required in order to assess the appropriateness of the conclusions made by the author(s).

Are there any conflicts of interest?

A conflict of interest highlights a personal circumstance that may potentially impact upon the action of the professional person or body. Research teams must make objective decisions and conclusions in the best interest of the patient, and conflicts of interest, such as financial gain, can cause certain studies to be conducted over others, creating a selection bias, thus highlighting significant results or adverse effects, and so on. Most papers employ an open disclosure form which highlights any and all conflicts of interest that may be present, and what actions have been carried out to ensure these do not affect the work conducted.

4.6 CV STRUCTURE

The all important CV should be included in your portfolio and must simultaneously house all of your most important and relevant content – while also being easily scannable by an interviewer, so that they can quickly appraise each section of your achievements/accomplishments. Your CV therefore needs to be highly organised with clear and concise headings. The following is an example CV structure that you can use to begin organising your CV.

General advice:

1. Place clear headings justified on the left
2. Place numbered listings or bullet points for publications, achievements, etc.
3. On the right-hand side have dates such as year clearly visible for each qualification, job, prize, audit, etc.
4. There should be no breaks in the timeline of your CV. Each period of time since entry into medical school should be accounted for.

CV structure

1. **Summary of personal details:** Placed in the header: Name, address, email and contact number
2. **Professional statement:** A brief paragraph of who you are and a synopsis of your career thus far and what your future road map is. This should at the least outline your desire to pursue a surgical career and to gain a place on a core surgical training programme as a step toward achieving that goal.
3. **Employment history:** e.g., FY1 in General Medicine, Name of Hospital, Area, Name of consultant. Start with your most recent job first and work backwards.
4. **Academic details:** This should include your GCSE and A Levels, degree(s), institution and level of achievement. Make honours, distinctions and merits clear in this section e.g. MBBS (Hons).
5. **Honours and prizes:** It is always impressive to place your prizes early in the CV. Give succinct but appropriate details that make it clear what the prize was for and to what level of competition was it involved, e.g., elective prizes awarded within year group of medical school, international prizes for research, academic prizes determined within year group.
6. **Publications:** This should include the title of the paper, the authorship on the next line with your name highlighted in bold followed by the citation of the article as it appears in publication or on PubMed, e.g., *Title of paper* First Author, **Your name,** third author et al Annals of Medicine and Surgery, 2014; 3(2): 41.
7. **Oral presentations:** Your oral presentations should follow a similar format with the title of the presentation first, authorship and then name and location of where the presentation took place. Place your name first and in bold if you presented the work.
8. **Posters:** Your poster presentations should follow a similar format with the title of the presentation first, authorship and then name and location of where the presentation took place. Place your name first and in bold if you presented the work.
9. **Audits:** Your audits should be organised with the title of the audit first followed by authorship. Below this you should have a statement that explains whether the loop of the audit cycle was closed, the gold standard used and whether any change to clinical practice was made.

10. **Elective details:** This is particularly helpful if you were involved in a surgical elective. Include the surgical specialty, institution/hospital and country. State also your consultant/supervisor and what the outcome from the elective was.

11. **Leadership roles:** This is an important section that should include the roles you have had that demonstrate your leadership qualities, e.g., foundation year representative, captain of sports team, medical society president, etc.

12. **Teaching:** This section must only include formal teaching sessions that you have conducted. State the name of the teaching session and the title that you had e.g. surgical teaching fellow. The name of the teaching module delivered e.g. Year 3 mock OSCEs and the institution/hospital.

13. **Courses:** The name of the course completed, institution are important here. Include taster sessions, specialty choice or study modules here also.

14. **Languages spoken:** Increasingly important in the multicultural and diverse environments we now work in. It is impressive if you are fluent in several different languages.

15. **References:** These are most often the same references that you submitted for the core surgical training application, but do not have to be. Include at least two recent supervising consultants with full name, address, email and contact numbers as well as their roles and specialties.

4.7 LEADERSHIP AND MANAGEMENT

You are likely to have been involved in several different activities that demonstrate your leadership and management qualities. You will require each of these in full measure. Many candidates feel they need to emphasise solely their ability to stand apart as a leader, when in clinical practice the majority of care is delivered in a multi-disciplinary team environment.

'Can you give examples of what makes a good team player?'

The important qualities of working in a team include consistency and reliability across all tasks that are undertaken. Working towards a goal that is in keeping with the rest of the team, and not just your own. Having a sense of responsibility and initiative to act without requiring regular prompts from a senior or team leader. Being able to adapt to a given environment or situation. An example of this is remaining on the wards to complete tasks and not taking every opportunity to attend the theatre. This reduces the burden of ward tasks on other colleagues, and ensures there is a fair rotation for other colleagues who may be interested in attending the theatre also.

'Can you give an example of when you played an important role within a team?'

During my rotation in trauma and orthopaedics, I acted as the translator between the surgical team and a patient who was visiting with their family from overseas. The patient had suffered a neck of femur fracture which required an operation, and I was able to translate the important and salient information to the patient and their family, as well as relay their concerns to the surgical team. This helped to expedite the history, examination and relevant investigations. I remained a constant relay not only for the surgical team but also the physiotherapists, the geriatric team and the nursing staff who were involved in the patient's care.

'What is the difference between a leader and a manager?'

In my experience, a leader tends to set the goals or objectives that need to be achieved by the group. They command the decisions that will lead to the group achieving these goals, and have the overall responsibility for the success of the team, as well as the failures or problems that they may face. A manager is more often involved in ensuring the group has the capacity to meet the specified objectives. This may involve a redistribution of resources, raising of red flags or worrying situations. A consultant is a good example of a team leader, whilst the lead in a PBL session is an example of a good manager.

4.8 NHS E-PORTFOLIO

It is always tempting to simply print your entire portfolio in readiness for the interview, without further analysis. However, it is wise to review your assessments and reflections since candidates have been asked specific questions about their e-portfolio, including work-based assessments and reflections. Once you have separated your portfolio into CBDs, miniCEXs and DOPs, and so on, read through these to refresh yourself regarding the various cases that you might be assessed upon. In particular, be able to recall significant events that you have reflected upon, important CBDs and miniCEXs. It is also important that you know your portfolio well enough to quickly turn to any given page and present the relevant section to the interviewers.

Based on our surveys of foundation doctors, the overriding opinion of the e-portfolio tends to be negative, however, in theory it is a valuable training tool. Most trainees would agree that having a more senior colleague overview their clinical history and examinations, as well as procedures, is helpful with constructive feedback. The prevailing reason for negative feedback against the portfolio appears to be the nature of the feedback given. Consultants and other senior members more often than not do not have the time to critique a history or examination properly, or indeed spend 20 mins going through a case in full detail. This is purely due to logistics and other clinical commitments, rather than anything else. The CBD, miniCEX and DOP assessments tend therefore to be sent to those team members who are most likely to complete them and/or give good feedback, thus bypassing the constructive feedback that may help improve skills.

Despite these opinions, there are limited other ways in which a deanery can adequately measure the progress of a trainee, and therefore these assessments are still employed to monitor your training as a core trainee, and indeed in higher training also. Other than CBDs, CEXs, multi-source feedback and DOPs, you should be aware of the other assessments that you will be undertaking as a core trainee to demonstrate your awareness and maturity as a prospective trainee:

- **Procedure-Based Assessments (PBAs):** These assess the trainee's technical, operative and professional skills for a given procedure. For most surgical specialties, every procedure has a PBA assessment that allows you to determine how well you performed a given facet of the operation, e.g., draping the patient, adequate response to complications, etc. This is to test global domains in surgery, but also specific technical skills for the individual operation. They are very useful in monitoring progress through a series of procedures, as well as serve as a guide to the operative steps involved

- **Assessment of Audit:** Audits are formally evaluated, highlighting their importance at core training level. The presentation of an audit is reviewed by your supervisor and then appraised based on relevance, standards, methods, results, implementation, etc.

  - **Observation of teaching:** This promotes formal teaching and allows for recognition and feedback of teaching outside of informal arenas, such as bedside teaching, etc. This is at present an optional work-based assessment, and although with increasing emphasis upon teaching, it is a valuable assessment to have in your portfolio. Linking this assessment and its importance to the teaching evidence in the portfolio (you present at your core surgical interview) will instantly raise you above other candidates.

We have compiled a list of questions that you may be asked regarding your NHS e-portfolio, use them with your portfolio to refer to relevant CBDs, miniCEXs, etc.

1. What do you think about the NHS e-portfolio system?

2. Can you give an example of a stressful clinical situation that you reflected on? Did reflective practice help you at the time? Has it helped you looking back on the experience?

3. Can you give an example of the most helpful case-based discussion that you have had?

4. How would you measure progress in surgical training?

5. Do all the deaneries have the same criteria when assessing you at ARCP?

4.9 RESEARCH

Evidence-based medicine

The concept of evidence-based medicine advocates the use of the best evidence obtained from the very best medical research to formulate the guidelines, protocols and the basis for treatment of patients. Among the plethora of research, studies and articles, one must retain the ability to appraise, evaluate and discern between credible and acceptable research findings from those that are not valid. This is the process of critical appraisal, which evaluates amongst many other properties the quality of evidence and study design. In order to appreciate the importance of research in clinical medicine and also to tackle questions that may be posed in the portfolio section of the core surgical interview, we have summarised some research concepts to complement the statistics section of this guide.

'How is the quality of evidence assessed?'

The critical appraisal of research may be assessed under the following categories:

1. Hierarchy of study design
2. Study quality
3. Consistency
4. Directness/applicability
5. Recommendations

1. Hierarchy of study design

There are various types of study design which are important when assessing the credibility and power of a given research paper. These studies can be graded in the following list in descending order of power:

A. Meta-analyses and systematic reviews
B. Randomised controlled trial
C. Cohort studies
D. Case control studies
E. Surveys
F. Case reports

Meta-analysis

This powerful study tool analyses several primary trials (most often randomised control trials) to evaluate the quality of evidence for a given research question. The combined analysis of primary studies can support the outcomes of the original studies since a given medication, or intervention, may only have a small impact when studied in isolation. A clear disadvantage here are the heterogeneous study designs and methods used across various studies.

Randomised controlled trials

A randomised controlled trial (RCT) allocates all candidates taking part in the study, through a fair and random process, into different groups, typically the treatment group and the placebo group. Candidates ideally should be as similar to one another as possible, so that any changes are as closely related to the intervention as possible. Once allocated, these groups are then analysed over a specific period of time to measure a given outcome, or effect, established at the very beginning of a trial. RCTs are considered to be at the top of the hierarchy of research studies, though this is always dependent on the clinical questions that is being investigated.

Advantages

1. Accurate and astute investigation of a single, measured variable
2. Reduces bias through randomisation, and comparing groups that are similar to each other
3. Prospective studies
4. Allows for meta-analyses to be performed

Disadvantages

A. Expensive
B. Time consuming and demanding
C. Exclusion criteria may limit investigations or application of outcomes

Cohort Studies

A cohort study analyses participants based upon their exposure to a given stimulus such as a toxin, medication and so forth, and reviewed over time to measure a given outcome, such as disease development. The groups should ideally be matched (age, gender, socioeconomic background, etc.) to allow for unbiased comparisons. Given the prolonged time any given exposure can take to cause an outcome, groups are typically followed over many years. Cohort studies can not only establish causal links such as 'Does smoking cause lung cancer?' but also demonstrate dose–response relationships such as 'Are heavy smokers more likely to develop cancer?'

Case control studies

In contrast to cohort studies, a case-control study takes patients already suffering from a given state of interest, such as disease. These patients are then matched to similar candidates without this condition and then investigated to identify a potential exposure that may be contributory. This may involve ascertaining the past medical and social history, or even having patients recount previous exposures. Case control studies are most useful for investigating rare conditions. As with any study, case control series are subject to bias and weaknesses. Poor definition of what the disease or condition is, with subsequent misallocation of participants, can cause disastrous impacts on the outcomes of the study. Similarly, case control studies cannot establish any causal relationships – only risk associations.

Survey

A survey attempts to answer a specific clinical question through the investigation of a representative sample of participants at a single point in time. This investigation can take a number of forms such as completing questionnaires, undergoing investigations or examinations.

Case Report

A clinical case report typically shares the history, investigation and management of a rare presentation with the aim of learning from the disease diagnosis, management, investigation or general discussion and so on. Several case reports can be used to produce a case series, which can be used to demonstrate a common denominator, such as an adverse drug reactions. Despite ranking low in the hierarchy of studies, case reports are still considered valuable in the information they provide, which is often missed in higher power studies. They are also of course much easier to conduct, publish and understand.

2. Study quality

A poorly devised and conducted randomised control trial can easily be overruled by a well-designed and executed cohort study. The study quality is just as important as the type of study conducted since factors such as randomisation, confounding factors, bias, blinding, and so on all have a substantial impact on the ultimate outcomes and conclusions of a study.

3. Consistency

A given clinical question will often have several studies and publications attributed to it. The consistency of findings is important, as any publication that goes against the trend of previous valid findings will instantly be viewed with suspicion and caution.

4. Directness and Application

All outcomes and results of research studies must be placed within a clinical context, and the impetus behind any study should always be in the bigger picture, with the aim to improve patient care and clinical practice.

Recommendations

Related to application, the recommendation of a clinical study can be in favour of, or detract away from a given intervention, investigation or treatment. It is important to note that however compelling the results of a study may be, the ultimate decision lies with the clinicians and practicing bodies to make decisions and create guidelines. It is therefore essential that a general understanding of research is gained.

5. OFFERS AND CLEARING

Offers usually follow approximately one month after the initial interviews. Candidates may then choose to accept their offer, hold for an upgrade or reject the offer. If you accept an offer, you will then automatically be withdrawn from any other national recruiting process that you may have been involved in. Candidates may hold an offer for a given period if they are waiting to hear back from other specialties. There is also an offers upgrade system where you can choose to be upgraded automatically to a higher preference, if it becomes available at a later stage. Upgrades are not guaranteed, and you will have to accept an offer first before taking part in the upgrade process.

The clearing process exists to place candidates who have achieved a nationally appointable score to vacancies within the country. Following clearing, a round 2 application process may take place, but is subject to the decisions made by national recruitment. In 2014, there was no round 2 clearing process for England. Candidates therefore had to email LETBs in N. Ireland, Wales and Scotland individually for the remaining core training posts that were still available.

The core surgical training application represents the first significant application for formal training in surgery. We have experienced first hand the daunting task that lies ahead in making a successful application to core surgical training. In this guide, we have included the very best advice and experiences that ensure you will be able to rank as a top candidate for core surgical training, and apply for the jobs you want. At first glance, do not be discouraged by the stations and questions we have included. Ensure you have enough time to read and re-read this guide, and to practise with colleagues. You will improve exponentially and – on repeating the stations and questions within this guide – be in the best possible position before you attend your interview.

Core surgical training is a fantastic platform to begin your formal surgical career and we hope each and every one of you makes a successful application.

Thank you for using this guide, and good luck!

INDEX

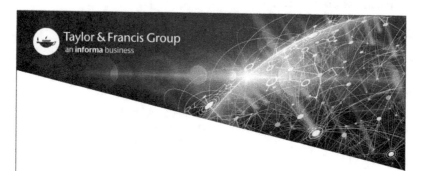